DR GRAY'S
WALKING CURE

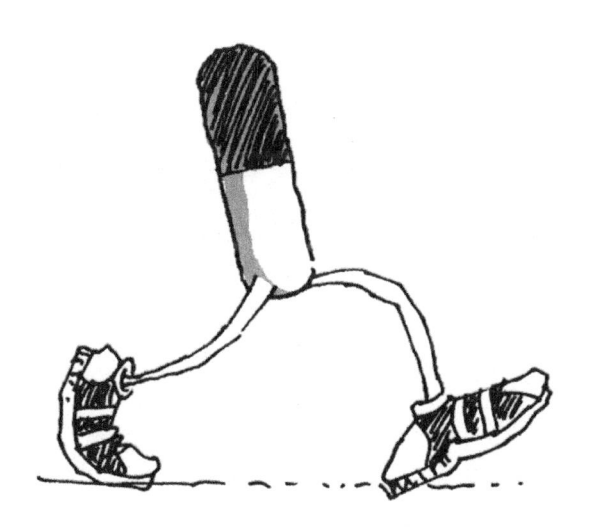

DR GRAY'S WALKING CURE

MUIR GRAY

OFFOX PRESS
OXFORD

DR GRAY'S WALKING CURE
www.drgrayswalkingcure.net

First published 2025

This book is copyright. All rights are reserved. Apart from any fair dealing for the purpose of private study, research, criticism or review, as permitted under the Copyright, Designs and Patents Act 1988, no part of this publication may be reproduced, stored or transmitted, in any form or by any means, without the prior permission in writing of the publishers. Enquiries should be emailed to Offox Press Ltd, books@offoxpress.com

© J.A. Muir Gray 2025

Muir Gray hereby asserts his right as set out in sections 77 and 78 of the Copyright, Designs and Patents Act 1988 to be identified as the author of this work wherever it is published commercially and whenever any adaptation of it is published or produced.

British Library Cataloguing-in-Publication Data
A catalogue record for this book is available from the British Library.

ISBN 978-1-904202-28-8

Although every effort has been made to ensure the accuracy of the advice in this publication, the responsibility for its use rests with the individual reader. Neither the publishers nor the author can be held responsible for the consequences arising from the use of any information contained herein.

Illustrations © 2025 by David Mostyn
Cover Design by Elaine Leggett
Typesetting by Bicester Publishing Ltd

CONTENTS

Introduction	ix
Foreword	x

CHAPTER 1: The benefits of walking are enormous	1
Extra steps, necessary steps, or vital steps?	1
Think small, act big	2
Brisk walking is key	3
But don't forget counting the steps	4
Gentle walking is much better than sitting	5
The start of your journey	6
Your height, weight, and Body Mass Index (BMI)	6
Your resting pulse rate	7
Your age	7
The Fitness Gap	8
Your medical conditions, if any, or many	10
Taking the first steps	11

CHAPTER 2: The risks of walking are tiny	12
Foot problems are the only internal problems	12
Bears, Ticks, Dogs and Cows	13
Risks from other road users	14
Falls	15
Use of a walking stick	16
Use of Nordic walking poles	17
Use of a wading stick	17
Pollution	18

CHAPTER 3: Stopping sitting	19
The dangers of sitting	19
Different types of sitting	20
How much do you sit?	21
The benefits of standing	22
Light intensity exercise	23
Down with sitting, up with standing – at home	24
What everyone should do	24
Down with sitting, up with standing – at work	25
If you are not the boss	25
If you are the boss, take the lead	26

CHAPTER 3 (continued)
Take action every day — 27
Take action every weekend — 28

CHAPTER 4: Enticing young people to walk more — 29
Childhood obesity is increasing — 29
What parents can do — 30
Start a campaign — 30

CHAPTER 5: Planning and implementing your walking revolution — 32
So what should I do? Count Steps, or Time? — 32
Measure how far you walk now — 33
Start walking more — 34
Use bus-stops as your stopwatch — 35
Finding time for brisk walking — 36
  Brisk walking for commuters — 36
  Brisk walking for home-workers — 36
  Brisk walking for office tasks — 36
Finding the motivation for brisk walking — 37
Keep a record of your walking — 37
The benefits for people who use wheelchairs — 37

CHAPTER 6: Walking to stay healthy and live better for longer — 38
Walking to improve fitness — 39
The 'Walking Plus' Programme — 39
  Increasing strength — 41
  Increasing suppleness — 41
  Increasing stamina — 42
  Increasing skill — 42
Walking to reduce the risk of serious disease — 43
  Reducing your blood pressure — 44
  Reducing your cholesterol — 44
Walking to get younger — 45
Walking to reduce your risk of dementia — 46
Walking to feel better — 47

CHAPTER 7: Walking for better weight control — 49
Getting your energy balance right — 50
Do your genes matter? — 52
Measuring food by steps and seconds — 53

Don't just eat less, eat differently	54

CHAPTER 7 (continued)
The weight loss drugs and walking programme	54

CHAPTER 8: Walking therapy — 56
Preventing the combination of disease and loss of fitness	57
How walking exerts its therapeutic effect	58

CHAPTER 9: Walking prescriptions for common conditions — 60
The origin of activity therapy	60
Digital support for activity prescribing	61
Walking therapy for people with COPD (Chronic Obstructive Pulmonary Disease) and asthma	61
Walking therapy for people with heart disease	63
Walking therapy for people with high blood pressure	64
Walking therapy for people with Type 1 diabetes	64
Walking therapy for people with Type 2 diabetes	65
Walking therapy for people with arthritis	66
Walking therapy for people with intermittent claudication	68
Walking therapy for people with osteoporosis	68
Walking therapy for people with neurological disease: stroke, multiple sclerosis, and Parkinson's disease	69
Walking therapy for people with cancer	71
Walking therapy for people who are depressed and/or anxious	73
Walking therapy for people with severe mental health problems	75
Walking for people affected by dementia	76
Walking for people who want to increase their ability	77
Social prescribing and the need for walking prescription	78

CHAPTER 10: Try different types of walking — 80
Talking walking	80
Meeting walking	80
Green walking	81
Awe walking	82
Silly walking	82
Phoning walking	83
Reading walking	83
Learning walking	83

CHAPTER 10 (continued)

Thinking walking	83
Sporty walking	84
Mindful walking	84
'Slow Ways' walking	85
Imaginary walking	85
Virtual reality walking	86
Race walking	87
Dog walking	87
Wellbeing walking	88
Purposeful walking	88

CHAPTER 11: Generating political action for the walking revolution — 89

The new environmental challenge	89
Mobilising political action	92
The Ramblers	95
Sustrans	96
Living Street	96
Take action to increase your wellbeing	97
Website of great organisations supporting walking	98

Introduction

In my fifty years in the NHS I have seen many wonderful treatments and technologies come into practice: chemotherapy, hip replacement, and transplantation to give three examples, but research has also revealed the vital physical and mental effectiveness of exercise. The Chief Medical Officers of the United Kingdom have consistently recommended thirty minutes of exercise, such as brisk walking daily, as a means of preventing, delaying, or even reversing the modern epidemics such as stroke, dementia, Type 2 diabetes, and obesity. We have also had the Report from the Academy of Medical Royal Colleges with the astonishing title *Exercise, the Miracle Cure*. Increasing the amount you walk is the simplest way to take the Miracle Cure, needing no special equipment apart from a raincoat now and again.

The evidence about the preventive benefits of exercise is now both overwhelming and accepted, but too many people identified at being at risk of disease are only getting a prescription for pills, not for walking. The position is even worse for people who already have one, or more than one, long-term condition; only a minority of them are prescribed anything other than pills. Pills are very important and often necessary, but they are not sufficient. A drug prescription for people with a long-term health problem should always be accompanied by an activity prescription, and the easiest to prescribe is to walk more. There is no obstacle to walking more as the Ramblers have shown by ensuring blind people can enjoy their walks.

This book is part of my campaign to inform and encourage people to walk more, and for the NHS to prescribe walking both for prevention and for treatment. It is of vital importance in helping you not only to live longer, but also to live better for longer, both mentally and physically.

I wish to thank John Churchill, Tom Futter, Gordon Galsworthy, Elaine Leggett, David Mostyn, and Jackie Rosenthal for their patience and skill in the production of this book.

Muir Gray

Foreword

Muir Gray is undoubtedly one of the most creative minds in British medicine today. The flow of ideas from such a mind is a complex and unpredictable process. The genesis of this book can be traced back to a cold February evening in 2006. Muir, an avid karaoke exponent, was performing at a pub in Oxfordshire, The Bleeder's Arms. The song he had selected, The Walk of Life by Dire Straits, was mispronounced by the karaoke compère as The Walk for Life. In his mind, Muir turned over this error and from it emerged Dr Gray's Walking Cure.

The potential benefits of walking as a regular form of physical activity are unequivocal in promoting overall health and wellbeing, reducing the risk of cancer and heart disease, as well as combating the modern epidemic of overweight and obesity, itself a risk factor for cancer, heart disease, high blood pressure, diabetes, and other illnesses.

Muir Gray assembles the evidence, sets out walking schedules for individuals to follow, covers what few risks there are, and makes the public health case for action to get the country on the move.

He presents the evidence, facts, figures and information in a highly informative and interesting way. Memorable quotations and whimsical references add to this small book's accessibility.

This book is another winner from Dr Gray's prolific pen. If you are in rural Oxfordshire and want to pop into The Bleeder's Arms for a pint and a pie, make sure you take 10,000 steps to earn them. If you pick the right night, you may even see Dr Gray's wiry frame (BMI 19) twitching and tracing the air-guitar chords to a 1970's rock classic (Some dance to remember, he dances to forget).

Sir Liam Donaldson
Former Chief Medical Officer (CMO) England

CHAPTER 1

The benefits of walking are enormous

'The walking cure is of vital importance. We spent seven million years of our history walking and now, all of a sudden, we are sitting down. This is having a profound effect on our health.'

James Levine, *Professor of Medicine, The Mayo Clinic*

Human beings are not designed for sitting. A major evolutionary trend has resulted in the ability to walk yet we now live in a world in which walking is not easy. It is still easier in the UK than in the USA, where sidewalks have disappeared in many urban areas and walking is reserved for the gym or golf course, both reached by car. For many people, however, even in the UK, driving is essential for work, either because public transport is poor or because a car is needed for the job itself. For these and other reasons, we walk less than previously, and less than we need to for good health and wellbeing. But everyone can walk more – that is, more than the minimum necessary for work or daily life – and the benefits are enormous.

In this book, I present the Walking Cure, that is, how you can put walking at the centre of your life and improve your health and wellbeing. By making small adjustments to your day-to-day life, you can add at least one or two thousand – or, better still three thousand – preferably brisk steps to your present daily average. The effects of such a change will help to control your weight, improve your health, and make you feel, and look, better. No sweat, no running, no lycra – just walking for a better life.

Extra steps, necessary steps, or vital steps?

Let us imagine you get through your day with, on average, 8,000 steps – some days more, some days less. You will get a health bonus if you walk 9,000 steps a day, a double bonus if you walk 10,000 steps, and a huge health bonus if you have walked for 30 minutes with moderate intensity. But how are these steps best described?

They could be described as 'extra steps' if they are in addition to the steps you take to work, or while you shop, cook, clean, and get through your daily life, but the word 'extra' sounds as though these steps are optional, superfluous, or unnecessary. In one sense, this is true; they are unnecessary to fulfil the tasks you need to do, but they are necessary for your health.

Think small, act big

You spend one-third of your life asleep, and always will. You spend at least another third in the workplace, either at home, or in an office or other work environment. Some people spend more than eight hours a day working, and an hour or more commuting; in addition, some people need to spend time looking after family, and/or doing housework, shopping, and cooking before and after they have finished paid work.

That leaves one-third of your life for 'other stuff'. Although retired people have more freedom, they still need to think about how to manage the time they have available because they will benefit more than people of working age from increasing the amount they walk.

The Covid pandemic dramatically affected people's lives, not only with a shift to homeworking, but also with a considerable decrease in physical activity, due in part to the emphasis on 'social distancing', particularly during the first lockdown. An Age UK analysis of the impact of the Covid pandemic found that:

> *'27% of older people (around 4.3 million) can't walk as far since the start of the pandemic.'*

By contrast, in the Active Lives Adult Survey November 2020-21 Report, Sport England found that of the activities showing growth before the pandemic, only walking continued to see numbers increase – up 2.4 million to 24.2 million people in 2021.

These national figures, however, hide considerable differences among different groups in society. For instance, people from the most deprived areas and from certain ethnic groups tend to walk less.

To adapt your lifestyle to the 21st century environment, you need to identify or create small amounts of time in which to walk briskly:

- 10 minutes a day will give you 1,000 Steps daily
- 20 minutes a day will give you 2,000 Steps daily
- 30 minutes a day will give you 3,000 Steps daily

In 2004, the Chief Medical Officer (CMO) for England, Professor Sir Liam Donaldson, distinguished doctor and Newcastle United fan, published the first Chief Medical Officer's (CMO's) report on physical activity and public health, in which it clearly stated that:

> *'A total of at least 30 minutes a day of moderate–intensity physical activity on five or more days a week reduces the risk of premature death from cardiovascular disease (heart attacks and stroke) and some cancers, and significantly reduces the risk of Type 2 diabetes, and it can also improve psychological wellbeing.'*
>
> At Least Five a Week. Evidence on the Impact of Physical Activity and its Relationship to Health. Department of Health, April 2004

In 2019, the four CMOs of the UK reinforced this message as did the CMO for England in his 2023 report, in a set of *Physical Activity Guidelines* in which they emphasised that:

> 'Each week adults should accumulate at least 150 minutes (2½ hours) of moderate–intensity activity (such as brisk walking or cycling).'

As we shall be using the adjective brisk increasingly throughout this book, you need to understand what we mean by it.

Brisk walking is key

There are many ways of walking (as described in Chapter 9), but there are two main types of walking your body needs to learn: regular walking and brisk walking. In the 2004 CMO's report, there is a description of moderate intensity exercise, and brisk walking fits this description.

- an increase in breathing rate
- an increase in heart rate to the level where the pulse can be felt

The 30 minutes of moderate–intensity physical activity necessary for health improvement can be built up in spells of 10 minutes, for example, in three 10-minute walks, instead of catching the bus for short journeys. Even 10 minutes a day will generate a health bonus if you are able to make it a regular feature of your life.

- 1,000 steps = half a mile
- 1,200 steps = 1 kilometre
- 1,500 steps = 60 calories

Ten minutes a day is easy to find, either during work time or other time, or, even better, during both. Even 10 minutes of extra walking every day is sufficient for the basic dose of the Walking Cure when it becomes part of daily life because it adds up. For example:

- 10 minutes = 1,000 steps
- 5,000 steps x 50 = 250,000 steps in a year (allowing for a couple of weeks when you are not able to find time)
- 250,000 x 4 = 1 million extra steps in four years – an Olympiad!

Therefore, with this small adaptation you can become a walking millionaire. A million steps equals:

- 500 miles or 800 kilometres
- 20 marathons
- 40,000 calories
- 80 litres of petrol

Of course, if you can manage to walk 2,000 or 3,000 extra steps a day instead of driving, all these figures double or treble, respectively. Imagine what an impact it would have on the environment if one million people walked an extra 3,000 steps a day for four years:

- 240,000,000 litres of petrol would not be used!

But don't forget counting the steps

Although there has been a shift from recommending 10,000 steps a day to an emphasis on achieving 30 minutes of moderate-intensity exercise such as brisk walking, step-counting remains important. It is easy, and objective. For people who are not walking very much to begin with, it is helpful initially to focus on the need to increase the step-count.

In a major review in *The Lancet* of the factors that determine how independent a person will be in their 60s, 70s, 80s, and 90s, the first three words of the article were 'Every step counts'. In another major review of the evidence published in *Lancet Public Health*, it was concluded that adults taking more steps per day have a progressively lower risk of all-cause mortality and the benefit 'can be seen at levels less than the popular reference of 10,000 steps per day.'

Gentle walking is much better than sitting

Although we are keen to promote brisk walking, we recognise this activity is beyond the capability of some people, at least to start with, because they have been sedentary for years. In the 2019 *Physical Activity Guidelines* by the four Chief Medical Officers, it was emphasised that:

> *'Prolonged sedentary behaviour is associated with many poor health and functional outcomes in older adults. There is emerging evidence that for inactive older adults, replacing sedentary behaviour with light-intensity activity is likely to produce some health benefits.'*

Any type of walking is better than sitting, as indeed is standing (described in Chapter 4), but brisk walking is still important for people in their 80s and 90s, and even people who cannot stand can now use Motus VR technology and a plastic plate on which they can slide their feet to walk virtually along the Great Wall of China or the town they grew up in, chatting to others as they do. There has also been tremendous progress in the development of equipment to support people. The legendary Zimmer Frame is still used but there are now a number of variants. Some have a seat, some have a wheel and brakes, and these are sometimes called Rollators. Type 'walkers for seniors' into Google to see the range. As the target of 1,000 extra steps a day may be too demanding for people over 80 years of age, unless they are already averaging 7,000 or 8,000 steps a day, we recommend the following starting targets:

- For people aged 80-89 years: 500 extra steps daily
- For people aged 90-99 years: 200 extra steps daily
- For people aged 100 years and over: 100 extra steps daily

Remember that the person may be walking slowly with a Rollator, but if the respiratory rate is faster than the resting rate the walking may be classified as being brisk.

Once these starting targets have been achieved, more ambitious ones can be set.

The start of your journey

Unfortunately, the starting point for any journey is where we are in the present moment, no matter how we might feel or look. The good news is you can start the Walking Cure whatever your age, wherever you live, whatever you do, and irrespective of whether you have health problems. There are, however, four factors that need to be considered:

1. Height and weight
2. Resting pulse rate
3. Existing health problems (if any)
4. Age

Your height, weight, and Body Mass Index (BMI)

The amount of fat a person has can be measured in several ways. You can look in the mirror and be honest. You can measure your waist. You can ask an expert to measure the fat under your skin using special pincers, the most reliable method scientifically. You can calculate your Body Mass Index (BMI), using a formula that relates your weight to your height. For this, you need to:

- weigh yourself, naked, in kilograms
- measure your height in centimetres
- put these measurements into a BMI calculator

It is easy to find the NHS BMI healthy weight calculator by searching Google. Once you have entered your measurements and calculated your BMI, compare your BMI with the standards drawn up in the US National Institutes of Health (NIH) guidelines:

- A BMI of less than 18.5 = underweight
- A BMI of 18.5 -24.9 = healthy range
- A BMI of 25-29 = overweight
- A BMI of 30 or over = obesity

Walking can help you to reduce and control weight (see Chapter 7).

Your resting pulse rate

Your resting pulse rate is the number of heart beats per minute at rest; the lower your rate, the fitter you are. Knowing your resting pulse rate is a useful baseline against which to judge whether you are walking briskly. Your resting pulse rate is a relatively easy measurement to take. Your pulse can be readily located in two places, as follows:

1. Place your index and middle fingers on the side of your neck in the soft hollow area beside your windpipe
2. Hold your arm straight with the palm facing upwards, and place your index and middle fingers on your wrist at the base of your thumb

Always use your fingers to find your pulse, not your thumb. If you can't find your pulse at first, move your fingers around a bit.

Once you have found your pulse, measure it for 30 seconds, then repeat the measurement 1-2 minutes later. Add the two figures together and divide by two to get your average resting pulse rate.

If you are finding it difficult to take your resting or walking pulse rate, the sense that you are breathing a little more quickly but can still carry on a conversation is a good enough test of briskness.

Your age

There is no upper age limit for walking. In fact, the older you are the more you have to gain from walking. In the 2004 CMO report, it was stated that:

- *'The beneficial effects of physical activity on cardiovascular disease, Type 2 diabetes and obesity, are also evident for older people.*

- *Regular lifestyle activity is very important for older people for the maintenance of mobility and independent living.*
- *Strength-training exercises can improve muscle strength, which is important for tasks of daily living such as walking or getting up from a chair.*
- *Physical activity – particularly training to improve strength, balance and co-ordination – has also been found to be highly effective in reducing the incidence of falls.*
- *Physical activity can help improve the emotional and mental wellbeing of older people. It is associated with reduced risk of developing depressive symptoms and can be effective in treating depression and enhancing mood.'*

In 2019 *Physical Activity Guidelines*, the four CMOs reinforced this message.

Although Alzheimer's disease remains a disease that it is impossible to prevent or treat, promising developments are taking place. However, it is not the only cause of dementia. There is now strong evidence that the risk of dementia can be reduced significantly, and that physical activity is one way of reducing the risk. Physical activity has both a direct and an indirect effect because it prevents or reverses other risk factors, notably Type 2 diabetes and high blood pressure. The normal biological process of ageing is relatively unimportant.

It is essential to understand what is happening as we live longer. The ageing process starts at about 20 years of age – from then on, it is downhill all the way. The good news is that the rate at which we decline can be slowed for almost everyone. Overall decline is a combination of decline due to ageing and decline due to inactivity:

Rate of decline = decline due to ageing + decline due to inactivity

The Fitness Gap

The difference between how able you are and how able you could be is called 'The Fitness Gap' (Figure 1).

In later life, the level of fitness may determine whether a person can climb a flight of stairs to reach the toilet in time. The Fitness

Gap can be closed at any age by walking plus simple exercises to improve strength, suppleness, and skill.

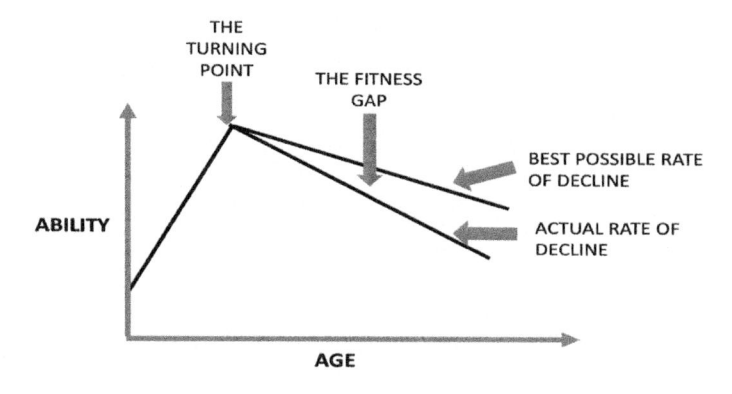

Figure 1: The rate of decline in fitness and The Fitness Gap

Many changes observed after the onset of disease are not due to the disease process but to an accelerated loss of fitness (Figure 2). This loss of fitness occurs principally because some people think that rest is best, whereas we now know that exercise is the 'miracle cure', and by closing the fitness gap people can improve, retain, or regain the level of ability needed to perform a vital task like getting to the toilet in time. This will be discussed in more detail in Chapter 8 on Walking Therapy.

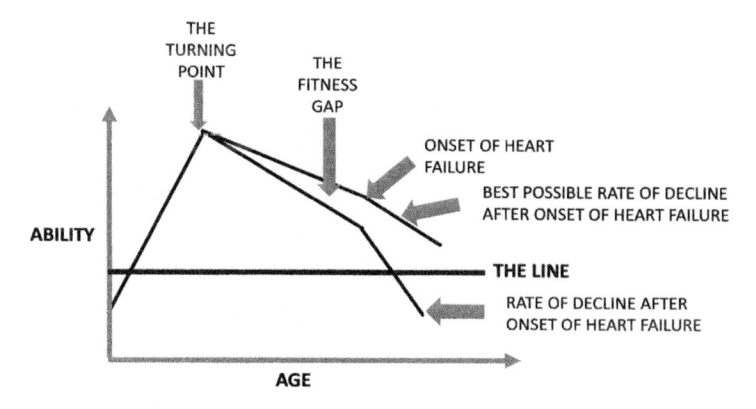

Figure 2: The rate of decline in fitness after the onset of disease

The aim for everyone should be to reduce the fitness gap and stay above the fateful line below which a person is not able to get to the toilet in time. The evidence is that no matter how old you are, or how many conditions you may have, you can close the fitness gap and live longer better. Walking plays an important part in closing the fitness gap.

Your medical conditions, if any, or many

> *'Walking is as close to a Magic Bullet as you'll find in modern medicine. (If there was a pill that could lower the risk of chronic disease like walking does, people would be clamouring for it.'*
>
> Jo-Ann Manson, Professor of Medicine, Harvard University

In a 2015 report from the Academy of Medical Royal Colleges entitled *'Exercise – the Miracle Cure'*, it was emphasised that exercise is an effective treatment for all the common long-term conditions.

Many people, including doctors, worry about the risks of exercise for people with long-term health problems. If you have a long-term health problem that you are concerned might be made worse by exercise, consult your doctor or nurse before increasing the amount you walk. In 2021, however, in a Consensus Statement from Sport England and the Faculty of Sport and Exercise Medicine on the risks of activity for people with health problems, it was concluded that the benefits of exercise were greater than the risks, as expressed in the title of the Consensus Statement – *'Benefits Outweigh Risks'*.

If you have one or more long-term conditions, you have a greater need for walking than if you do not. You may not be able to manage 1,000 extra steps a day, but every 100 steps you take will improve your health and reduce the harmful effects of disease, which so often come from inactivity. Furthermore, other people, who may think it is better for you to be in a wheelchair rather than lending you an arm or buying you a stick to help you walk, need to change their perspective.

If you have one or more long-term health problems, walking is beneficial because it may help:

- reverse the condition, especially if combined with a change in diet. It also supports and maintains weight loss, which will help reverse high blood pressure and Type 2 diabetes
- reverse the loss of fitness that often occurs after the onset of disease as many people become less active, not because of the effects of the disease but because other people, with the best of intentions, start to do things for them

The importance of walking as a therapy is only now becoming generally accepted by the medical profession because the evidence is strong that there is no upper age limit and no limit on the number of conditions that a person may have and still benefit from walking.

Taking the first steps

You can start by measuring how much you walk now and make a plan for walking more. Alternatively, you can just start walking more, but to do this you will want to be reassured not only that the benefits are massive, but also that the risks are tiny, the subject of Chapter 2.

CHAPTER 2
The risks of walking are tiny

No human activity is free from risk. Even if you were to stay in bed for the rest of your life, you would run the risk of fatal venous thrombosis. Moreover, there is no such thing as 'safe' healthcare; all healthcare carries the risk of harm or adverse effects as well as the potential for benefit.

All human activity, therefore, is a matter of balancing risks, in this case, balancing the risks of walking against the risks of not walking. Compared with other activities, the balance of risk for walking is highly favourable, and the risks that do exist can be minimised.

Exercise therapy, therefore, has a highly favourable balance between the probability and size of benefit, and the probability and size of harm, with only a few small incidental risks.

The risks can be divided into two types:

1. Internal risks – potential adverse effects in your body
2. External risks – potential adverse effects resulting from the environment in which you walk

Foot problems are the only internal problems

The foot consists of an intricate assembly of bones that create an arch, supported by tendons stemming from the calf muscles, which extend across the arch.

The most common internal risk from walking is a foot problem, such as a painful heel. Strong calf muscles can lower the risk of foot problems. The risk of foot problems can also be reduced by wearing the right shoes.

A good selection of walking shoes is now available. If you are building walking into your working day, you may prefer to wear shoes that are good for walking – that is comfortable after walking a mile – but do not look as if they have been specially designed for walking. For men, many manufacturers now make shoes that look good and are well designed, making urban walking more pleasurable. I wear trainers for urban walking and meetings, and am often approached by men who tell me they would like to do the same! Well, why don't they?

High-heeled shoes do not necessarily cause problems. In a well-designed study of women with arthritis of the knee, it was found that wearing high-heeled shoes did not increase the risk of arthritis in the knee.

> *'It is very unlikely that prolonged wearing of high-heeled shoes represents a risk factor for symptomatic osteoarthritis of the knee in women.'*
>
> Dawson, J et al. (2003) An investigation of risk factors for symptomatic osteoarthritis of the knee in women using a life course approach. Journal of Epidemiology & CommunityHealth 57; 823-830.

If foot problems do occur, consult a registered podiatrist. Podiatrists are one of the most valuable, but often under-rated, of the clinical professions. Your podiatrist may also call on the skills of an orthotist, who make special insoles to rebalance the bones of the foot.

Bears, Ticks, Dogs, and Cows

The external risks of walking depend on the environment in which you are walking. In his book, *A Walk in the Woods*, Bill Bryson describes his fear of being attacked by bears on the Appalachian Trail. Pepper sprays are useful, according to Stephen Heurer in his book, *'Bear Attacks: Their Causes and Avoidance'*. Fortunately, the risk of bear attacks is not high in the UK, but the risk of adverse effects from another animal, the tick, is increasing. The tick is not an insect but a member of the spider family (known as an arachnid) that sucks blood from its host, and in the process injects into the host's bloodstream bacteria from the *Borrelia* family, which can cause Lyme disease. Lyme disease is becoming more common in the UK as the ambient temperature rises. Advice from The Ramblers about minimising the risk of tick bites is shown in Box 1.

Box 1: Minimising the risk of tick bites

- Wear trousers and long-sleeved shirts and keep cuffs fastened and trousers tucked into socks
- Wear shoes or boots rather than open sandals
- Use insect repellent: DEET or Permethrin can protect against ticks for several hours
- If you find a tick, remove it quickly, preferably with a specially designed tick removal tool. These are better than household tweezers as they avoid the risk of squashing the tick and releasing fluids into your skin. In an emergency you can use a thread of cotton looped around the tick's mouthparts, which you then pull steadily upwards
- After your walk, carefully brush all clothing and examine yourself for ticks. Pay special attention to their favourite feeding places: the backs of knees, around the groin, under the arms and, especially on small children, the hairline and scalp

The behaviour of some dogs can pose a problem. When faced with a barking dog, the best advice is to stand still until the owner appears. If the owner does not appear, it may help to turn away and ignore the dog. Walk away, do not make eye contact, speak to, or touch the dog. Always keep your hands in your pockets.

Cows with calves can be far more dangerous than bulls, and need to be given a wide berth.

Risks from other road users

'The main hazard for walkers, runners, and cyclists is an increased risk of unintended injury from a motor vehicle crash.'

At Least Five a Week. Evidence on the Impact of Physical Activity and its Relationship to Health. Department of Health, April 2004

Being hit by a car is a risk on both country and city roads, and pavements. At night, a reflective bandolier reduces this risk, but some people do not want to wear them, and a light-coloured jacket or coat is a sensible compromise.

Although it is good to see more people cycling, the practice of pavement cycling is hazardous for people who are walking, and in recent years this has been compounded by the risk of being hit by a scooter.

Walking in busy streets is as good for your health as walking in quiet streets, but air pollution, particularly from transport-generated particulate matter and nitrogen dioxide, especially in urban areas, is a growing problem.

Walking with friends is also a good way of increasing safety and security.

> *'Respondents who had good street lighting, trusted their neighbours ... having access to sidewalks, and using malls, were associated with regular walking.'*
>
> Addy, C. L. et al. (2004) Associations of perceived social and physical environmental supports with physical activity and walking behaviour. American Journal of Public Health 94: 440-443.

Conversely, people who live in poor-quality or threatening environments are less likely to walk – another reason why people in the most-deprived areas are at higher risk of many diseases. Although women who go out to work are very active during the day, doing two jobs, one at their place of employment, the other at home, it can be difficult to combine exercise and work. The results of a survey carried out by BUPA and the magazine *Top Santé* showed that:

- 52% of the women interviewed found it 'totally impossible' to fit exercise into the day
- 80% of the women interviewed said they never walked to work

Falls

Falls are serious events, which sometimes cause a fracture. The risk of falling is greater on uneven ground and when ambient light is poor. Most of the serious falls occur in the home, but many falls occur outdoors, in part due to the poor maintenance of pavements. The risk of falling is increased by leaves on the pavements in the autumn, and frost and snow in the winter. Consider how often the roads are free from frost due to gritting by councils, whereas the pavements are glassy with ice because councils claim they do not have the resources to clear the pavements. In some cities, such as Chicago, a different culture prevails, and people are required, to clear the pavement in front of their dwelling, and to help a neighbour if they are unable to do clear their own section of pavement.

- Walking not only improves strength and skill but also reduces the risk of falling.
- Walking also helps to prevent bone loss (osteoporosis), only some of which is due to the ageing process, and thus reduces the risk of having a fracture if a fall should occur.

Use of a walking stick

The probability, or risk, of falling can be further reduced by using a walking stick, the advantages of which are shown in Box 2. People who are unsteady, or who have already had one fall, should use a stick. After the age of 80 years, probably everyone should use a stick.

Box 2: Advantages of using a walking stick or pole

- Less stress on hips and knees
- Easier to recover balance following a trip or stumble, therefore reducing the risk of a fall
- Gives a good rhythm to walking
- Reduces pressure on hips and knees when walking downhill
- Increases the amount of energy used, and two-pole walking, also known as Nordic walking, significantly increases the amount of energy expended

---

Use of Nordic walking poles

> *'Just the fact that they are using their arms more, through a greater range of motion than normal, means they are increasing calorie expenditure. Add poles, and they burn 20% more calories.'*

> John Pocari, Professor of Exercise Physiology,
> University of Wisconsin

Nordic walking is recommended as an effective form of exercise therapy, with no adverse effects. For many people, a Nordic pole is a great walking aid. They are used most often by people walking in the countryside rather than in the town or city – but why not use them in urban environments?

- Look at the website for Nordic walking (www.nordicwalking.co.uk)
- There are local groups with leaders who can introduce newcomers to this form of walking
- There are excellent books on the subject, such as *Nordic Walking* by Malin Svensson, and *The Complete Guide to Nordic Walking* by Gill Stewart

Use of a wading stick

On the first day of the Platinum Jubilee celebrations the Queen appeared on the balcony at Buckingham Palace with a walking stick that looked higher than usual, more like a shepherd's crook than a conventional walking stick. On the final day of the celebrations, she emerged with the walking aid that became her hallmark in later life: Prince Philip's wading stick. A wading stick is designed to help fly fishermen keep their balance on the uneven bed of a rapidly flowing salmon river. It is longer than a walking stick, the height of a Nordic pole, with a V-shaped grip at the top made from the natural branching of a strong twig or antler, and is weighted at the foot to increase stability.

Pollution

Although there is now much less smoke pollution from the combustion of coal, air pollution in urban areas from traffic has become a hazard in Britain, particularly from particulate matter and nitrogen dioxide. The risks to respiratory and cardiovascular health are real, but smaller than the risks from not walking; on balance, the benefits of walking outweigh the risks of air pollution to the lungs, because the risks of inactivity are far greater than the risks of walking. Some inactivity is necessary. Sleeping well reduces your risk of dementia, but there is one type of inactivity that is both dangerous and avoidable, and that is sitting, the focus of Chapter 3.

CHAPTER 3

Stopping Sitting

The famous illustration below, depicting the evolutionary path of Homo Sapiens, shows a progression from moving with the support of four limbs, through a stage when we relied on our forelimbs for steadiness when running, to a semi-erect followed by an erect posture. And then comes the slump into a chair, a dangerous position for our health and wellbeing.

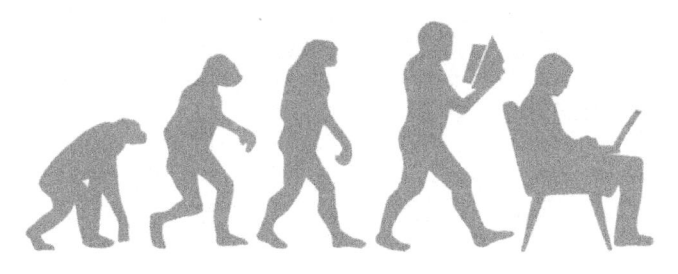

The dangers of sitting

The first important review of the adverse effects of prolonged sitting appeared in August 2011 when the American Journal of Preventive Medicine published a set of articles on *'The Science of Sedentary Behavior'*, which was followed by a systematic review in March 2012.

In one of the articles, the authors' focus was the need to have an internationally agreed measure of 'high sitting time', which was also becoming a growing problem in 'low-and middle-income countries'.

The principal article in this set was the first systematic review of all the research on sedentary behaviour since 1996. It was concluded that:

> *'There is a growing body of evidence that sedentary behavior may be a distinct risk factor, independent of physical activity, for multiple adverse health outcomes.'*

The findings of subsequent systematic reviews have reinforced this conclusion. In a review of 43 observational studies of television viewing and other sedentary behaviours, it was concluded that:

> *'Prolonged TV viewing and time spent in other sedentary pursuits is associated with an increased risk of certain types of cancer.'*

In two further reviews, it was found that sitting is not only associated with an increased risk of cardiovascular disease and Type 2 diabetes, but also with increased mortality.

In recent years, there has been increasing use of the slogan 'Sitting is the new smoking', and the Harvard Medical School's Special Health Report *Walking for Health* emphasises the importance of what they call 'Sitting Disease':

> *'Our society is by and large a sedentary one, where people spend far more time sitting than they did in previous generations: an average of 13 hours a day versus 3 in a true agricultural society, and that's a problem. The latest research shows that too much sitting may be more dangerous than smoking. It is now associated with 34 chronic diseases or conditions, including heart disease, diabetes, some types of cancer, back pain, depression, and possibly even premature death, according to 18 studies that involved over 800,000 people in the past 16 years.'*

So, there is a new epidemic. We could call it Hyper-Sitting Syndrome (HSS). It seems to be different from WDS – Walking Deficiency Syndrome – although the two conditions often occur together and both need to be tackled.

Different types of sitting

Any type of sitting has adverse health effects, but some types of sitting are worse than others, particularly for your core strength, namely the strength of your spinal, abdominal, back and neck muscles. For most people at work, the demands of the keyboard and the computer screen result in poor posture, with not only an increased risk of heart and vascular disease, Type 2 diabetes, and some cancers, but also increased risk of low back, shoulder, and neck pain, and of repetitive strain injury (RSI).

Sitting on a sofa is even worse, and most people's TV viewing is done from a sofa. Although designed for relaxation, the sofa induces the worst of all sitting positions.

Research evidence indicates that driving is worse than sitting on a sofa, probably because of the stress involved in driving. Although it is possible to get your posture right when sitting in an individually adjustable driver's seat, too many people sit with their spine curved forward. For many people, commuting by car is a fact of life, often for an hour or more each way, sometimes combined with the need to drive during working hours. People who commute by car must try to build three 10-minute brisk walks into their daily routine, and the people who love people who need to commute by car should encourage this! Moreover, employers should build brisk walking into their employees' working day, as part of their duty towards employee health and wellbeing and because they can be assured that employees will work better with walking breaks as well as coffee breaks.

How much do you sit?

The key issue is how much do you sit and how can you sit less?

Homeworkers in particular face problems, usually because the work they do tends to involve sitting. Consequently, their routine may be limited to moving straight from the bed to the breakfast table and then to the desk, or it may be shortened to clearing the breakfast table and switching on the laptop, or to simply switching on the laptop and maintaining a stream of hot buttered toast and marmalade. At least people who use public transport to get to work must walk to and from the bus stop or railway station and, if they are lucky, they may have to stand during the journey.

All standing is good, and standing on a bus, train, or tube is very good. It uses more energy, strengthens the leg muscles, and maintains and increases balancing skills, all of which are part of 'Walking Plus', our walking programme that primarily improves stamina, augmented by additional exercises to improve strength, suppleness, and skill. While sometimes it may be necessary to sit on public transport, in general it is best to try to stand.

The benefits of standing

The benefits of standing are only now being recognised, including the increased energy expenditure.

- Sitting or sleeping = 1 calorie per minute
- Standing = 2 calories per minute
- Walking = 4 calories per minute
- Brisk walking = 6 calories per minute

Big deal! Standing for one minute requires one more calorie than sitting. In Scotland, however, they have a proverb, 'Mony a mickle maks a muckle', which loses a lot in translation, but means 'Many little things add up to a big thing'. For instance, if you had a job that required you to sit for eight hours a day and you changed that to standing for eight hours a day for 47 weeks a year, the effect would be equivalent to running 69 marathons.

Although no-one is going to change from being completely sedentary to standing all the time, in a review of the changes needed to combat the problems caused by 'the sedentary office', scientists at the University of Minnesota, led by Professor Christopher Reiff, concluded that:

> *'For those occupations that are predominantly desk-bound, workers should aim to initially progress towards accumulating two hours per day of standing and light activity (light walking) eventually progressing to a total accumulation of four hours per day.'*

Some people's jobs require them to stand all day, such as retail staff, assembly line workers, catering staff, and library assistants. Prolonged standing has its own problems, including aching muscles, pressure on the hip, knee, and ankle joints, back problems, and damaged feet. Those whose work involves prolonged standing, such as hair stylists and dentists, and must also hold their head and shoulders in a particular way, can increase the stress on certain muscles and joints. Many derive benefit from Pilates or Tai Chi, which should be offered.

Light intensity exercise

Much of the research has been focused on exercise of 'moderate–intensity', which has led some people to ignore or discount exercise of light intensity. James Levine, a British doctor working at the Mayo Clinic Research Institute, has shown the importance of light activity, especially as we do so much of it. In his book entitled *Get Up! Why Your Chair Is Killing You and What You Can Do About It*, he introduces the concept of NEAT, an acronym for 'non-exercise activity thermogenesis', namely, *'the calories that people burn when they are moving when they are not sitting'* (Levine's italics). An example of this would be standing rather than sitting.

Replacing non-stop sitting at work with standing is a topic of growing interest, especially with the recent increase in homeworking due to the impacts of the Covid pandemic.

Ergonomics is the study of how people work, and a team in the ergonomics lab at Cornell University has developed a useful formula for people who sit non-stop at work. In every half-hour (30-minute) period, people need to:

- Sit for 20 minutes
- Stand for 8 minutes
- Walk about for 2 minutes, even if it is only to the printer

To replace sitting with standing, you don't necessarily need to invest in an expensive standing desk, simply change the way you, and perhaps your manager, think to get you off your bottom (see Box 3). Whatever equipment you decide to use to enable you to stand while working, it is important to ensure that it is at the right height to prevent backache and poor posture when standing.

When standing to work on a computer or laptop, it is important to align the height of the screen with your eyes and position the keyboard at an appropriate level for your hands, arms, and shoulders. Adjustable workstations and lecterns are available that can be put on top of your existing desk or table.

> **Box 3: Useful books about the impacts of sitting**
>
> 1. *Is Your Chair Killing You? A Healthier You in as Little as 8 Minutes a Day* by Kent Burden
> 2. *Sitting Kills, Moving Heals* by Joan Vernikos
> 3. *Deskbound: Standing Up to a Sitting World* by Kelly Starrett

Standing has many advantages over sitting. People's posture is almost always better when standing, although some people do stand badly, with their head jutting forward, and their arms folded in front of them. To achieve a good posture when standing, you need to aim to make the crown of your head as the highest point.

Down with sitting, up with standing – at home

If you are a homeworker, although it is relatively easy to build standing into your day, you may need to be creative. For instance:

- While watching TV, stand up for the advertisements, or stand up and down 10 times when the advertisements are on. Remember not to use your hands to push up from the chair or sofa. (The benefit from this exercise is increased if it is done with a 3kg weight in each hand. If you do not have any weights, you could use a 1kg bag of unopened sugar in each hand!)
- Watch the News, or football, on TV standing up; it is only in the last 20 years that everyone has had to sit down when attending a football match
- Watch concerts on TV standing up, as though you were at the Proms. If you go to a concert or festival outdoors you would probably stand, if only to prove you are still young and cool.

What everyone should do

Irrespective of whether your job involves prolonged sitting or standing, everyone needs to stretch, ideally for 15 minutes during the day. It might be easier to do 10 minutes in the morning and 5 minutes when you can manage it during the day, or when you get home (see Box 4), but every minute of stretching you do counts.

> **Box 4: Stretching exercises for people who sit a lot**
>
> - Stand straight, arms bent at shoulder height, and try to get your elbows to meet behind your back. Don't worry, no-one can do it, but this stretches the chest muscles. Repeat 10 times every hour
> - Keep standing straight, then turn your chin to the left as far as you can, and hold for a count of 10, now turn to the right and hold for a count of 10. Repeat five times every hour

The book written by Diana Moran, the Green Goddess, and Muir Gray titled Sod Sitting, Get Moving -Getting active in your 60s, 70s and beyond has good advice from that dangerous phase of life -Retirement.

Down with sitting, up with standing – at work

If your job requires you to sit at work for four or more hours a day, you need to take action, and the action you are able to take depends on your environment. For most people in office jobs that involve sitting at a computer or speaking across a counter while seated, there is scope for increasing the amount of time to stand. Taxi and lorry drivers, for example, and those who need to sit for 8 or more hours a day must take exercise: brisk walking for 10 minutes three times during the working day, together with the stretching exercises described above. Almost all London taxi drivers have got the message and now exercise before or after work.

If you are not the boss

If you are an employee, you may need to convince the boss of the benefits of building standing into the working day. It would be a misguided boss who would not allow their team to do something that improves morale and reduces repetitive strain injury, sickness absence, and early retirement, but there are some misguided bosses around.

Well-designed standing desks are now available that enable the height to be adjusted to the height of the person typing or writing.

They are expensive, however, and may allow the boss to plead poverty. If you read or write a lot in your job, a lectern with a sloping surface will enable you to read and write at eye level and they are not expensive.

The Golden Rules governing standing to work are shown in Box 5.

Box 5: Standing to work – The Golden Rules

- The screen should be at eye level
- The keyboard should be lower, as though you were sitting
- Your feet should be slightly apart
- Occasionally lift one foot then the other to reduce tension on the hamstrings, and the muscles at the back of the thighs

---

It turns out that Scrooge (in *The Christmas Carol* by Dickens) was not such a bad employer after all: Bob Cratchit had a standing desk with a sloping surface and a little foot bar to raise one leg or another from time to time!

If you are the boss – take the lead!

Set an example by standing whenever you can. Introduce the activities suggested in Box 6.

Box 6: What you can do as a boss to increase standing and reduce sitting

- Hold standing meetings – they tend not to last as long, and people feel better
- Have one-to-one meetings and supervisions while walking. It is often easier to give feedback on aspects of performance that could be improved when side-by-side, rather than face-to-face
- Encourage team members to stand whenever appropriate
- Build standing and good posture into your team's culture, for example, by introducing stretching for suppleness, an important exercise for everyone
- Introduce lunchtime walks

Take action every day

Irrespective of whether you have done 10 minutes of strength and suppleness exercises before you leave home, it is important to encourage the team you work with to do the exercises developed from Yoga, Tai Chi, Pilates, and the Alexander Technique shown in Box 7 below. If one member of the team is an expert in any of these disciplines, ask them to lead.

Box 7: Exercises from Yoga, Tai Chi, Pilates, and the Alexander Technique

- Stand tall, against a wall. Stretch your neck and the crown of your head upwards, not forwards like a tortoise
- Put your arms along the wall, elbows and backs of hands touching the wall
- Take 20 deep breaths
- Slide your arms upwards like a windmill, keeping them on the wall, and hold this position for a count of 20. Repeat five times
- Step away from the wall and circle your arms slowly, brushing your ears as you take your arms backwards. Repeat five times
- Interlink your fingers and push your hands palms outwards, away from you, for a count of 10. Repeat five times
- Stand up straight, one foot well in front of the other. Bend the front leg as far as you can and hold for 20 seconds (you may also want to hold on to a desk with one arm). Do this five times with each leg

---

If no-one in the team is an expert, ask a teacher from one of the disciplines above to come in and lead a class occasionally.

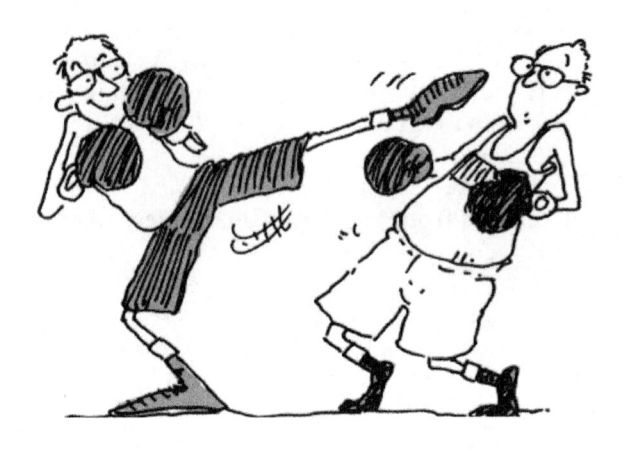

Take action every weekend

In early 2017, research demonstrated the benefits of being a 'weekend warrior', namely, someone who is not able to exercise during the working week but who takes exercise at the weekend. The conclusion was that some exercise is better than none, there is no 'magic' amount, and even the busiest person can find time to do at least some exercise. Weight control is only one health benefit from walking.

Walking should be considered as a therapy in its own right, which is discussed in Chapter 8. There is now strong evidence of its effectiveness as a therapy for many conditions. But before giving information on what you can do to renew and transform the part that walking plays in your life, we want to focus on one sub-group of society who need to walk more, and sit much less – young people.

CHAPTER 4

Enticing young people to walk more

The need for children and young people to walk more has never been greater. A combination of increased risks outside the home (road traffic, crime, and anti-social behaviour) and more attractions inside the home (a range of electronic devices and the TV) mean that children and young people are less active. Declining levels of activity have been found not only among girls, who drop out of school sport earlier than boys due to a combination of social attitudes and failure to appoint physical education teachers, but also in children under 5 years of age.

The short-term consequence is an increase in the proportion of children who are overweight, leading to an increase in the proportion of adults who are overweight. The level of physical ability at any stage in adult life depends not only on the rate of decline but also on the maximum level of fitness achieved during a person's childhood growth and development. Overweight, unfit children will become adults who have a higher risk of heart disease, high blood pressure, Type 2 diabetes, dementia, and cancer.

Childhood obesity is increasing

The results of a recent study in China showed that each hourly increase in watching television was associated with an increase of more than one percent point in the percentage of children who were obese.

Owing to increasing levels of obesity and decreasing levels of activity, Type 2 diabetes, which may be regarded as a complication of too many calories and too little exercise, is now being diagnosed in children, when previously it was a problem seen only in adults.

Solutions to the obesity epidemic in children and young people are numerous and complex, ranging from the feasible, such as a 'tax' on sugar, sugar-sweetened drinks, and ultra-processed foods, to the desirable but unrealistic, such as the abolition of the smartphone, tablet, and other devices. Walking in childhood can make an important contribution to health and wellbeing, not only because of its effect on bodyweight but also because of the mental health benefits.

Some measures to encourage walking can be taken by parents; others require social action.

What parents can do

Parents must provide leadership, but cunning is also justifiable! It is possible to park further from the intended destination than the closest possible car park to increase the amount the family walks. In unfamiliar cities, it is relatively easy to get away with this ruse, but it is more difficult in your home town. With younger children aged 2-10 years, distant parking is much easier.

Travelling by public transport can be made into an adventure, as a way of stimulating children to take more steps, without using the 'W' word!

Effective ploys include:

- Going to see interesting places, animals, or any leisure amenity that must be reached by walking
- Treasure hunts – organising things to search for around the corner or in the next street

Grandparents sometimes have the time, respect, and novelty value to do many of these things more effectively than parents, and it is often easier to get children walking more by engaging with other families.

Start a campaign

Encouraging children and young people to walk more, however, is difficult for parents to accomplish on their own, and social action is also needed to change the prevailing culture. Thus, the organised efforts of society can support parents and children:

- directly, by providing a range of activities at school and after school that promote physical activity
- indirectly, by changing the environment in which children and

young people spend their time. For instance, parental cars could be banned from a zone around the school so that children need to walk the last 500 steps to school

Intelligent Health is an organisation founded and led by Dr William Bird, a GP who was the originator of Health Walks. The organisation's aim is to make physical activity a way of life through the implementation of campaigns that have community benefits. Intelligent Health's mission is to create resilience and improve health by establishing a connection between people, between people and their communities, and between people and their environment. 'Beat the Streets' is one of Intelligent Health's programmes, comprising a real-life game played on streets and parks across a community. 'Beat Boxes' are attached to lamp-posts dotted around a town. Children aged under 11 years have a fob, and children and young people aged 12 years and over have a card, like a credit card. To get points, the children and young people must swipe the fob or card against a 'Beat Box'. The aim is to try to reach as many Beat Boxes as possible by walking, cycling, or scootering, although walking is the principal way of getting points.

Living Streets is a charity commited to making walking safer and more enjoyable. A major theme of its work is walking to school. There is a challenge for primary and secondary schools called WOW, and one feature of the challenges is winning a WOW badge, which pupils can get when they walk or wheel to school. Intergenerational walking is encouraged because some of their work is also focused on older people.

Let us now focus on your wellbeing and how walking can increase it, starting with a review of how much you walk now and by how much you want to increase it.

CHAPTER 5

Planning and implementing your walking revolution

So, what should I do? Count Steps, or Time?

In 2021, a systematic review of 1,017 good-quality articles measuring the effects of walking on 'community dwelling older adults' was published in the journal *Lancet Healthy Longevity* by a multi-national group of authors. The results of these papers were combined, and the conclusion was powerful:

> *'Higher physical activity and lower sedentary behaviour were most strongly associated with better chair stand test performance and lower body muscle strength, and least with falls and hand grip strength. Number of steps was most strongly and most consistently associated with clinical outcomes. Conferring to a wide array of positive outcomes, steps provide a clinically relevant target that shows practical ease. Future recommendations should promote steps regardless of ability, encouraging that some physical activity is better than none, or, as the present findings show, that every step counts.'*
>
> Ramsay, K.A. et al. (2021) Every step counts: synthesising reviews associating objectively measured physical activity and sedentary behaviour with clinical outcomes in community-dwelling older adults. *Lancet Health Longevity*

Over the last five years there has been lively debate as to what is most important:

- the number of steps (with 10,000 a day having been the magic number for years)? or is it
- the amount of 'medium-intensity exercise' taken (with at least 150 minutes a week of brisk walking being recommended)? or is it
- a walking rate of 112 steps per minute, as promoted by the authors of a paper in the journal *JAMA Neurology* in September 2022?

The message is clear: every step and minute counts, the brisker the better. So take action to walk your way to wellbeing.

Measure how far you walk now

Measure the number of steps you take for 7 days – see Box 8 for the devices you can use to count your steps.

Box 8: Devices you can use to count your steps

- Devices such as a Fitbit, Samsung Galaxy and Apple Watches – these measure several fitness variables
- Mobile phones – these measure mobility and ability. The iPhone has a focus on wellbeing and offers access to the Exi programme www.exi.life which suggests exercise programmes tailored to all the common conditions
- Apps for all mobile phone users, including the NHS Active 10 Walking Tracker, which measures how many minutes you walk briskly

---

Try not to increase the amount you walk just because you have started measuring, although you will feel the persuasive power of the tracking device, which makes you want to walk more from the moment you start using it.

Record your walking in a simple diary. Copy or photocopy the chart on the next page if you find this book too small to write in.

Day	Number of Steps	Number of minutes of brisk walking
Sunday		
Monday		
Tuesday		
Wednesday		
Thursday		
Friday		
Saturday		
WEEKLY TOTAL		
DAILY AVERAGE		

Start walking more

The target of 10,000 steps a day has been promoted for many years, but it may not always be possible for most people leading busy lives.

- A single parent taking a day off to look after a sick child might take 5,300 steps in the house, including a dash to the shops when a neighbour calls and can keep the child company for 40 minutes, but it is often simply not possible to squeeze in the necessary balance of another 4,700 steps before going to bed

- A sales manager, who has to drive to a conference in Manchester and returns at 11.30 pm having walked only 3,764 steps during the day, is not able to fit in the necessary balance of another 6,236 steps before midnight

In such circumstances, the focus needs to be on the amount of time spent brisk walking, not on the number of steps. The aim is to walk briskly for at least 30 minutes a day five days a week, although not necessarily in one session; it can be done in three 10-minute stretches or six 5-minute bursts.

Use bus-stops as your stopwatch

Extensive research shows that if you want to be sure of walking briskly for 10 minutes, you need to walk the distance between only four bus stops or, to put it another way, to walk the distance between three more bus stops than the one at which you usually get on or off. As the distance between bus stops varies, if you want to plan your walking precisely and take the same bus regularly, you need to measure the amount of time it takes to walk another one, two, or three stops. As time spent on the journey to work is precious, you should try to walk at least one to three bus stops before getting on the bus. Most bus routes now display real-time information showing how many minutes will elapse before the bus is likely to arrive.

So you can calculate whether you have the time to squeeze in one, two, or three bus stops, equivalent to three, six, or nine minutes of brisk walking, before catching the bus. If the distance from one bus stop to another takes five minutes to walk rather than three, you may be able to achieve your 10 minutes before catching the bus. There is less stress associated with the homeward journey. You can either walk one, two or three stops before getting on or, if a bus arrives instantaneously, you can catch it but get off three stops early and add another 10 minutes brisk walking to your account. In the CMO's 2019 *Physical Activity Guidelines*, it mentioned 'getting off the bus a stop early and walking the rest of the way', but the recommendation should have been to get off the bus early by several stops, and not one.

Similarly, if you drive to work, you can park at a car park half a mile or more from the office, and thereby build brisk walking into your day that way.

The great enemy, however, is time, and how you manage it. To walk more, it is important to open little windows of time in your day. There is probably enough wasted time to do this, but sometimes it is difficult to convert wasted time into walking time, except at the end of the day.

Finding time for brisk walking

As everyone's lifestyle is different, each person must work out how best to adapt their life to ensure enough brisk walking is done. The basic principles are clear:

- Your physical and mental health will improve if you walk more than you 'need to' for the demands of your day-to-day life
- If done regularly, 10 minutes' brisk walking a day will be beneficial, but you need to aim for at least 30 minutes of brisk walking on at least five days a week
- Walking uphill is even better for your health – try to walk up at least 100 stairs a day instead of using the lift or escalator

Adapting your life to include brisk walking will be made easier if you download the NHS Active 10 Walking Tracker app onto your smartphone.

Brisk walking for commuters

Brisk extra steps can be taken while getting to and from work, for example, by walking between bus stops in the morning or at the end of the day. For many people, changing from commuting by car to commuting by public transport will be enough to meet the brisk walking target – set up and establish a routine of walking between at least two bus stops on the way to work, and four or five bus stops on the way home.

Brisk walking for home-workers

People who work from home should walk briskly for 15 minutes before they switch on their computer, and for another 15 minutes in the middle of the day. As home-workers lose the benefits of walking as part of their journey to work, it is important to build it into the working day.

Brisk walking for office tasks

- If you have a meeting with one person, make it a walking meeting, not a sitting meeting
- Make the most of your phone calls while walking – phone on foot, not on your bottom

Finding the motivation for brisk walking

To find the motivation for brisk walking, it can help to
- write down the reasons you want to walk
- find other people to walk with, for example join The Ramblers or find out from the local health centre if there is a Ramblers Wellbeing Walk in your area. If not, why not start one?

Keep a record of your walking

To maintain your motivation for walking, it helps to keep a diary as a record of success. The diary can be kept as a hard copy or online, where you can post photos of your walks on your platform of choice. You may want to use a Fitbit or a smart watch, but every mobile phone can now record how much and how briskly you walk, using one of the many health apps that are available. One good app is the Exi app, another is the app launched by the NHS called the NHS Active Ten app. It is very good for recording your minutes of brisk walking should be at least thirty minutes daily as part of your campaign to reduce your risk of disease and stay healthy, which is the subject of the next chapter.

The benefits for people who use wheelchairs

All the benefits described in this chapter are relevant for people in wheelchairs, apart from, obviously, strengthening of the muscles of the lower limb. People in wheelchairs who push themselves have significant impact not only on the strength of their core and upper limb muscles but by increasing their respiratory rate they are doing exercise of 'moderate intensity'. This means that they will experience all the benefits of risk reduction, weight control and feeling better that people who walk do. It is essential that pavements are kept in good order and that there are paths through woods which people in wheelchairs can use. The charity Living Streets has made the needs of this section of the population a high priority in their campaign to improve pavements, and get rid of pavement parking.

CHAPTER 6

Walking to stay healthy and live better for longer

Physical activity can cut the risk of developing coronary heart disease by up to a half. It can also lower blood pressure, relieve stress, and minimise the risk of stroke and diabetes. Walking is one of the easiest, most convenient and inexpensive forms of exercise.'

Sir Charles George, Formerly Medical Director,
British Heart Foundation

While horses evolved to walk on the thickened 'fingernail' of the middle digit of each foot (which is what hooves are), early humans developed the ability to walk upright and use the hand to grasp objects. One theory is that this would have been advantageous at a time when much more of the earth's surface was covered by water; walking on hands and knees is not much fun when water is four feet deep everywhere! This ability to walk on two legs and use our arms and hands for other tasks gave the early human an advantage over other animals.

It is important to be aware that early humans evolved to walk, not to run, as an article by Peter Arnold entitled '*Why running is not for people*' in the 2003 Christmas edition of the *British Medical Journal* emphasised:

'Imagine our primitive forebear trying to chase a small mammal over the uneven terrain. The four-legged beast could put one foot into a depression or onto a mound, yet balance on its other three legs. Our biped ancestor had only to put one foot wrong – and catastrophe: at best a stumble, at worst a broken ankle.'

Today's joggers and runners don't seem to want to acknowledge the fact that the human body is not built for running, an activity that sends shock waves along the lower limbs, but is instead built for walking, which does not cause shock waves along the lower limbs. In the last 100 years, the need to walk has been reduced or diminished by technological developments, such as the motor car, the lift, and the escalator. During this time, however, it has become evident that walking brings many other benefits than simply getting from A to B (see Box 9).

Box 9: The advantages of walking, especially brisk walking

- Prevents weight gain, contributes to weight loss, and maintains weight loss once it has been achieved
- Improves fitness
- Reduces the risk of serious diseases – heart disease, stroke, Type 2 diabetes, dementia, and some cancers
- Helps you to stay young or become as young as you were
- Increases wellbeing

Walking is the best type of physical activity to help you stay healthy, particularly if you have one or more long-term conditions. In Chapter 8 on Walking Therapy, we summarise the benefits of walking for people who have long-term conditions.

Walking to improve fitness

Exercise and fitness: what images are conjured in your mind when you read these words? Perspiration, lycra, and a fitness centre or gym?

Fitness centres and gyms promote the message that you need to join one to get fit, but that is not the case. The opportunities for becoming fitter are everywhere:

- On the pavement outside your front door
- Up the flight of stairs by the lift in the hotel
- Up the flight of steps beside the escalator in the shopping centre
- Regular use of these opportunities to exercise can improve fitness without a hint of lycra.

The 'Walking Plus' Programme

A person's level of fitness cannot be measured when they are sitting still. It can be measured only when a person gets active. As an individual's level of fitness increases, the difference narrows between their heart rate and breathing rate at rest, and their heart rate and breathing rate when they are active. Fitter individuals have greater resilience, that is a greater ability to respond to a challenge (see below).

Differences in heart rate and breathing rate for an unfit and fit person at rest and during exercise

Heart Rate	Unfit Person	Fit Person
At rest	110	70
After four flights of stairs	180	95
Rate of breathing		
At rest	16	14
Rate of breathing	30	17

Walking can increase your fitness effectively and efficiently. It is often said that walking is less effective than belonging to a gym or fitness centre, and that may be true if a gym member attends regularly – but how many people do?

- Of the whole population, only a small proportion can afford to join a gym or fitness club
- Of those people who can afford to join, only a small proportion do
- Of those people who are members, only a small proportion go regularly
- Of those people who do go regularly, most get there by car, and sometimes have a beer and a sandwich after exercise

Unless you live next door to the fitness centre/gym, if you walked briskly to the fitness centre then turned around and walked briskly home again, you would get as much exercise as you would if you drove there, exercised, and drove back home.

Although walking is excellent exercise with many benefits, it will not improve all four of the main aspects of fitness:

1. Strength
2. Suppleness
3. Stamina
4. Skill

To improve overall fitness, you need:

- the 'Walking Plus' Programme, namely, 30 minutes a day of brisk walking, which is a good way of increasing stamina
- at least 12 minutes a day increasing your strength, suppleness, and skill

Increasing strength

The muscles of the lower limbs are strengthened by walking. Walking also strengthens the muscles of the lower back, which can reduce the likelihood of back pain. To complement the benefits from walking of lower-limb muscle-strengthening exercises, it is also important to exercise the upper-limb muscles and the muscles in the body's core, around the spine and abdomen.

Nordic walking also provides excellent exercise for the upper body.

Increasing suppleness

Walking helps to maintain the suppleness and flexibility of the lower limbs, but because the act of walking rarely stretches the muscles and other soft tissues, it is not a particularly good way of improving suppleness.

Therefore, it is good to supplement walking with other exercises to improve your suppleness and reduce stiffness. No-one understands exactly what causes stiffness, but it could be caused by various factors including:

- arthritis
- ageing and the loss of elasticity in the tissues

You might find that your legs are stiff after your first long walk, especially if you do an hour of brisk walking, but this will soon pass. The best way of preventing stiffness is to take exercise more frequently. One of the many advantages of walking as a form of exercise is that it is not necessary to 'warm up' before starting nor is it necessary to 'warm down' after you have finished.

If you want to improve your suppleness, it may be useful to join an introductory class for Yoga, Alexander Technique, Pilates, or T'ai Chi. Attending such a course will give you exercises that you can, and should, perform every day, not only for your hips and knees but also for the suppleness of your shoulders, arms, and spine. This requires you to build a five-minute suppleness routine into your day and, as was the case for finding the time for extra walking, it is a matter of time management.

Increasing stamina

Brisk walking can increase your stamina. When you start you may find it difficult to do brisk walking for more than 1,000 steps, but as you walk more frequently, your stamina will improve.

It is often difficult, however, to measure improvements in stamina. You may feel less breathless when walking briskly or be able to walk briskly for longer, but that could be because you have slowed down. To maintain and improve your stamina, the best way to ensure you keep walking briskly is to walk against the clock. You could walk 1,000 steps and measure the time it takes. A more feasible approach, however, is to walk briskly for a constant distance, such as the distance between specific bus stops, or from your home to the bus stop, and make that your test track. At least once a week, walk the track briskly and measure how long it takes, preferably to the nearest second.

The best piece of equipment for increasing stamina is a flight of stairs or, better still, four flights of stairs. Death to lifts or they will be the death of you!

Increasing skill

> *'Physical activity programmes can help reduce the risk of falling, and therefore fractures, among older people.'*
>
> *At Least Five a Week. Evidence on the Impact of Physical Activity and its Relationship to Health.* Department of Health, April 2004

Ageing reduces the body's ability to cope with challenges. One of those challenges is lack of exercise. For instance, although you may remember the skill of how to ride a bicycle, your ability to balance on a bicycle worsens as you age unless you keep cycling. This effect of ageing may not seem relevant to walking because most people retain the skill of putting one foot in front of the other. However, the skills necessary to walking that are lost are more subtle, although equally important, skills such as:

- Judging how far to lift your foot to clear the kerb or uneven parts of a pavement
- Recovering your balance if you should stumble
- The more you walk, the more these skills are maintained, but you should also try other types of exercise that are good for balance such as dancing, be it Scottish country, ballroom, or ballet. Moreover, dancing has many social benefits which promote mental wellbeing, in addition to the physical benefits already noted.

The ability to develop new skills or improve co-ordination was until recently thought to be impossible for anyone over sixty, but new technology for measuring brain function has shown this to be untrue. It is true that we cannot create new brain cells, but new connections and circuits can develop at any age in what is called neuroplasticity of the brain.

Walking to reduce the risk of serious disease

The World Health Organization has estimated the percentage of the total burden of common long-term conditions caused by physical inactivity (see below).

Proportion (%) of various common diseases caused by physical inactivity in men and women

Disease	Proportion of disease due to inactivity (%)	
	Men	Women
Cardiovascular	23	22
Colon cancer	16	17
Type 2 diabetes	15	15
Stroke	12	13
Breast cancer	Not relevant	11

The benefits of physical activity are therefore considerable, whereas the risks are negligible and relatively unimportant.

Reducing your blood pressure

There is no reason why people with high blood pressure should not increase their physical activity by walking. In fact, people with high blood pressure are more in need of brisk walking than people whose blood pressure is not high. One of the direct effects of brisk walking is to reduce blood pressure.

> *'Moderate intensity physical activity is associated with reductions in both systolic (3.8mmHg) and diastolic (2.6mmHg) blood pressure.'*
>
> *At Least Five a Week. Evidence on the Impact of Physical Activity and its Relationship to Health.*
> Department of Health, April 2004

Walking, however, also has an indirect effect on blood pressure by reducing bodyweight – obesity is a major cause of high blood pressure which, in turn, is a major cause of stroke.

> *'The majority of studies report that those who do regular light to moderate activity have a lower incidence of stroke compared with those who do not.'*
>
> At Least Five a Week. Evidence on the Impact of Physical Activity and its Relationship to Health.
> Department of Health, April 2004

Reducing your cholesterol

Walking can help to reduce cholesterol levels. Although statins are highly effective drugs, unless an individual has the genetic condition known as familial hyperlipidaemia, for a clinician to prescribe statins as soon as raised levels of cholesterol have been identified gives the wrong message. Although statins do lower cholesterol, someone with raised cholesterol needs to recognise they do not have Statin Deficiency Syndrome but instead need to change their lifestyle by eating less and eating differently, such as adopting a Mediterranean-style diet with fruit, salads, fish, pasta, and olive oil, and by walking more. In addition, one of the side-effects of statins can be muscular pain, which can mean that some people will walk less.

Similarly, someone with Type 2 diabetes does not have Metformin Deficiency Syndrome, but needs to change their lifestyle, including by walking more.

Walking to get younger

It is important to understand what happens as we grow older. The ageing process starts at about the age of 20 years. From then on, it is downhill all the way; the good news is that for almost everyone the rate at which we deteriorate can be slowed.

The rate of decline = decline due to ageing + decline due to inactivity

The difference between how able you are and how able you could be is known as the Fitness Gap, described in Chapter 1. The good news is that the Fitness Gap can be closed at any age (Fig.3).

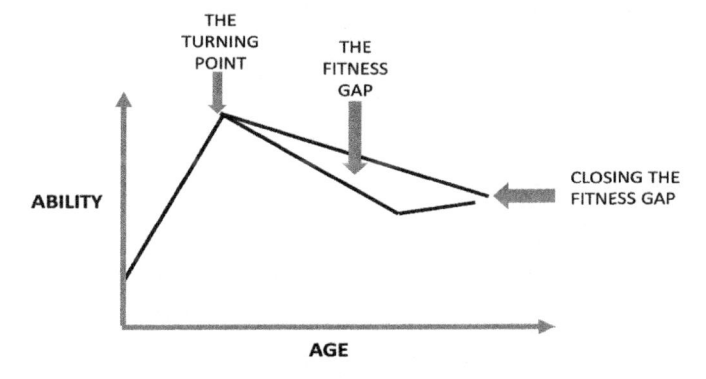

Figure 3: Closing The Fitness Gap

The 'Walking Plus' Programme, that is brisk walking plus simple exercises to improve strength, suppleness, and skill, will help you to close the Fitness Gap whatever your age. Closing the Fitness Gap restores your ability to the level you enjoyed 10 or more years earlier.

There is no upper age limit for walking: the older you are, the more you will gain from walking more, especially if you are walking briskly.

Walking to reduce your risk of dementia

Alzheimer's disease is the most common cause of dementia and cannot be prevented. Many people, however, have dementia from other causes, the commonest of which is any disease affecting blood supply to the brain. Therefore, walking, which reduces the risk of arterial disease, contributes to dementia prevention.

In 2004, Robert Abbot and colleagues in the *Journal of the American Medical Association* reported that walking can prevent the condition we all fear – loss of intellectual or cognitive ability:

> *'Findings suggest that walking is associated with a reduced risk of dementia. Promoting active lifestyles in physically capable men could help later life cognitive function.'*

In the same edition of the journal, a research group headed by Jennifer Weuve reported:

> *'Long term physical activity including walking, is associated with significantly better cognitive function and less cognitive decline in older women.'*

In the 2017 *Lancet Commission* on Dementia Prevention, Intervention and Care (LCDPIC), Gill Livingston and colleagues concluded that:

> *'Older adults who exercise are more likely to maintain cognition than those who do not exercise.'*

The 2017 *Lancet Commission* separately recommended the need to reduce blood pressure as well as prevent Type 2 diabetes, and walking contributes to reducing both these risk factors.

In 2022, the journal *JAMA Neurology* published the results of a study of 78,430 people in the UK (mean age of 61.1 years), in which Professor Borja del Pozo Cruz and colleagues from the Department of Sport Science and Clinical Biomechanics at the

University of Southern Denmark, concluded that:

> *'A higher number of steps was associated with lower risk of all cause dementia. The findings suggest that a dose of just under 10,000 steps per day may be optimally associated with a lower risk of dementia. Steps performed at higher intensity resulted in stronger associations [between walking and reduced risk of dementia]'.*

There is also evidence of the direct effects on brain tissue of walking. In a one-year study by Tarumi and colleagues of people with mild cognitive impairment published in 2019 in the Journal of Alzheimer's Disease, exercise training affected the way brain cells worked and connected with one another. Thus walking, particularly brisk walking, not only reduces the risk of vascular dementia by keeping the blood and oxygen supply to the brain healthy, but also affects the way brain cells work and their level of connectedness.

The practical actions you can take to reduce the risk of dementia are described in our book *Increase Your Brainability and Reduce Your Risk of Dementia*. These actions will also reduce your risk of becoming frail and help to prevent another condition we all fear – the need for social care.

Walking to feel better

Regular walking can make you feel better, as well as look better. There is evidence that people suffering from anxiety and/or depression can improve their mood by taking extra steps each day. Walking more can also help if you are feeling stressed. The beneficial effects of walking are partly due to:

- the distractions offered by a new environment – sitting at home surrounded by the same four walls is less stimulating than seeing what is happening while out walking, particularly walking in a green environment
- the release of chemicals called beta-endorphins, which improve mood
- the feeling of achievement from walking 1,000, 2,000, or 3,000 extra steps is good for self-esteem

Walking more can also help prevent or reverse the accumulation of fat, which affects most people and causes obesity, or WDS (Walking Deficiency Syndrome) as we prefer to call it, which is the focus of Chapter 7.

CHAPTER 7

Walking for better weight control

'The nature of human physiology is that it is extremely difficult, if not impossible, to maintain a healthy bodyweight with a low level of physical activity.'

Hill, J. (2004) Physical Activity and Obesity.
The Lancet 363:182

First, you need to decide whether you are overweight, which can be done in one of three ways:

- Measure your waist and compare it to what it was when you were thirty
- Calculate your Body Mass Index (BMI) – a formula that relates your weight to your height
  - Weigh yourself, naked, in kilograms
  - Measure your height in centimetres
  - Enter your measurements into an online BMI calculator such as the one on the NHS website
  - Now compare your BMI with the obesity league table
    - A BMI of less than 18.5 = underweight
    - A BMI between 18.6 and 24.9 = healthy range
    - A BMI between 25 and 29.9 = overweight
    - A BMI of 30 or more = OBESITY
- Finally, there is a wonderful invention known as a mirror which can help you decide whether you are overweight! Have a look and be honest.

Whichever method you used, what have you decided? Are you overweight or obese?

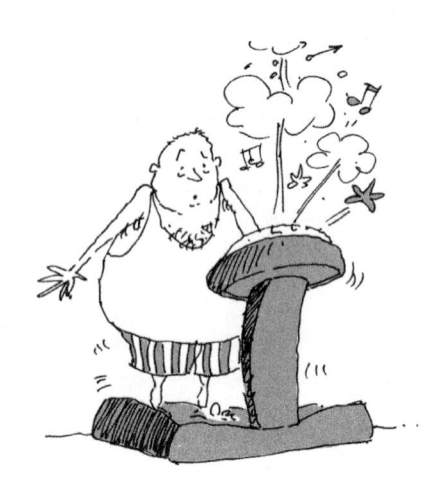

If you want to lose weight, combining walking with dietary change will help because walking increases the amount of energy you use, and burns calories. Even if you are not overweight now, it is important to take preventive action because modern life drives people remorselessly towards obesity. For a variety of reasons, we do a little less every year, and as such use a little less energy – we might get promoted, we become busier, or we simply give up the struggle. As a result, the average weight for both men and women increases with each decade lived, but it doesn't have to be that way if you get walking.

There is now, of course, a pill to accelerate weight loss and some people have found this helpful, but for long-term weight control, for example keeping the weight off after you have lost it, a plan to walk more, particularly to do more brisk walking daily, will help keep that weight off.

Getting your energy balance right

A human being needs energy to function, much like a car needs fuel to run. If you put more fuel into a car's tank than it will hold it will be blown back. In your body, however, the relationship between need and supply is not as well regulated. If we take in more energy than we need, the surplus is not rejected like the fuel from a full tank. It is converted into fat.

The presence of fat in your body acts as an energy store. If extra energy is needed, for example, when no food is available, the energy stored in the fat is released and used. Such challenges are less common in countries with developed economies, but unfortunately there are other circumstances that make the consumption of more energy than is needed all too easy:

- Food is readily available, and high-energy/high-calorie ulta-processed foods are relatively cheap
- Labour-saving devices have reduced the amount of energy we expend at work and home
- The car has reduced the amount of energy we need to expend to travel from A to B

It is mainly for these reasons, and not necessarily because people are overeating, that obesity is becoming more common. Most people who are overweight become so because, each day, they take in as little as 100 calories more than the amount they need.

- 1 biscuit = 100 calories
- 100 calories per day x 365 = 36,500 calories per year
- 36,500 calories = the total energy intake needed for 18 days

There is an obesity epidemic in the USA, and the UK is not far behind. Weight gain can be prevented by:

- A little more energy expenditure through exercise – walking would do the job very well
- A little less energy intake, by consuming fewer calories

In other words, weight gain can be prevented by a change in the energy balance:

> *'A little more walking (about 2000 additional steps) or eating a few less bites of food.'*

Hill, J. (2004) Physical activity and obesity.
The Lancet 363: 182.

Do your genes matter?

In 2016, the CMO of England at the time, Dame Sally Davies, made the focus of her annual report, the human genome, and devoted a chapter to 'Genomics and Obesity'. She emphasised that some people who are overweight become so not only because they take in more energy than they need but also, they have inherited certain characteristics that make it more likely that they will become obese.

- Some people are more efficient at converting surplus energy to fat
- Some people continue to feel hungry for longer after they have consumed enough food and therefore continue eating – they do not have a well-developed sense of satiety or fullness

Both these factors increase the likelihood that a person will become overweight, and there is no doubt that some people put weight on more easily than others. Being able to put on weight was an advantage until about 200 years ago, because people who accumulated fat in the summer were more likely to survive the winter.

Of course, the population does not fall into two separate groups of people but there is a spectrum, with some people who are very efficient at converting surplus energy into fat at one end and, at the other, people who can eat what they like and do not get fat. Most of us are somewhere in the middle of the spectrum. All of us, however, are subject to the law that if we consume more energy than we need on a regular basis, our bodies will convert that excess into fat.

Irrespective of your genetic make-up, you can control your weight by changing the balance between energy intake and energy output.

The Chief Medical Officer's report of 2016 recognised the contribution that:

> *'The genetic drivers of food intake and satiety have on obesity and weight-gain highlights the damaging and powerful effects of the current obesogenic environment, with its omnipresent stimuli encouraging consumption of high calorie foods.'*

In *The Story of the Human Body*, Daniel Lieberman, explains how we have a Neanderthal body in a post-Neanderthal world. By this, he means that our bodies evolved to live in a world where people had to be very active to find enough food to survive, a bit like being on a Bear Grylls survival course. We no longer need to be this active in order to find sufficient food, and our bodies are therefore no longer well adapted to our environment. Indeed, this mismatch between our body and the modern environment we now inhabit is a disadvantage.

Measuring food by steps and seconds

There are many ways of controlling your weight, but if you want to lose weight and keep it off, walking has an important role to play. Both Slimming World and WeightWatchers emphasise the need for walking as part of their solutions to weight loss. These programmes also have the added benefit of support and encouragement from other members of the group towards meeting your goal of losing weight and improving your health.

Although you may need to change your calorie intake to lose weight, you certainly need an increase in walking to keep your weight down. As calories don't mean much to most people, it is helpful to remember:

- 10 minutes of walking = 1000 steps = 40 calories
- 1,000 steps of brisk walking = 60 calories

A simple approach is to avoid all foods between meals that take more than 10 minutes of walking to burn off. It is unlikely that a person walking 6,000-7,000 steps a day will become obese eating only knife-and-fork dishes if each contains at least two portions of vegetables.

The foods to avoid are high-fat or sugary snacks and 'fast' food, which may be tasty but are:

- low in volume, that is, they can be eaten in five minutes, and do not satisfy the stomach for long, (sometimes referred to as satiety)
- high in calories and take at least 60 minutes to walk off the energy consumed
- full of chemicals because they are ultra-processed

Remember that 30 minutes of brisk walking five days a week for a year is equivalent to a weight loss of 4.5 kilograms or 10 pounds.

Don't just eat less, eat differently

There is now evidence that the lower rate of heart disease in southern Europe is not due to the sunshine but to the Mediterranean diet. This diet includes at least five pieces of fruit or vegetable a day, uses more olive oil and less butter, and omits biscuits and other high-energy low-volume snacks so beloved in the UK. Although the Mediterranean diet can include a glass of wine a day, alcohol-free days are good for your health.

There are many weight-loss/diet plans available, with more appearing every year. The NHS Weight Loss Plan is a 12-week plan with a free app. Keep it on your phone beside your NHS Active 10 app (also available for free from the Apple app Store or Google Play).

Weight control is only one health benefit from walking. Walking should be considered as a therapy in its own right, as there is now strong evidence of its effectiveness as a therapy for many conditions, which we summarise in Chapter 8.

The Weight Loss Drugs and Walking Programme (WLDWP)

One of the most significant drug developments of the last decade, indeed of the last fifty years, has been the development of drugs which are effective for losing weight. In 2025 there are three available but others will follow and they are effective in a short period of time. However people who have put on weight need to think long term and drugs alone is not the best strategy. The person who is prescribed such a drug should also be prescribed walking, aiming for 30 minutes a day of brisk walking which is equivalent of about 10lbs of fat a year, particularly if combined with a tasty diet based on the principles of the Mediterranean diet, and well described on the British Heart Foundation website.

Of course simply telling someone they need to walk more does not always lead to action. People need to be informed and encouraged and the benefits of the Walking Programme should be reinforced at every repeat drug prescription together with

- Information about local health walks
- Encouragement to walk with friends, in a green environment if possible
- Links to opportunities for sponsored walking, not to raise money for themselves but for a good cause like the Wildlife Trust

CHAPTER 8
Walking therapy

'The benefits of walking are countless.'

Lucy Knight (2007) Walking *For Weight Loss.*
The easy way to shed pounds and stay slim.
Kyle Cathie Ltd

In the last 50 years, there have been many medical miracles – new surgical operations, such as the hip replacement, new pain-free diagnostic investigations such as magnetic resonance imaging (MRI), and new drugs – all of which have increased the life-expectancy, and quality of life, for millions of people. The treatment of cancer, heart disease, arthritis, and many other conditions has been transformed.

Today, all doctors can also prescribe walking as a therapy, based on evidence from multiple research studies summarised in *Exercise – the Miracle Cure*, the 2015 report from the Academy of Medical Royal Colleges. The prescription of walking, and other physical activities, is known as 'social prescribing' or 'activity prescribing'.

Rest is the appropriate prescription for acute health problems, which range from a life-threatening heart attack to pneumonia. For long-term conditions, however, walking has a major contribution to make, not only to altering the course of the condition, but also to help the affected person:

- feel well
- regain ability lost in the acute phase of the condition
- increase fitness to a level greater than that before the onset of disease
- reduce the risk of other diseases – for example, that someone with high blood pressure might develop Type 2 diabetes

The role of walking is even more relevant after the impact of the – Covid pandemic, not only for those people who had Covid some of whom had experienced the common complications of 'long

Covid' – but also because of the effect of lockdown on everyone in the population, especially older people. In a 2021 report from the Department of Health entitled the *'Wider effects of Covid on physical activity, deconditioning and falls in older adults'*, it is estimated that an additional 110,000 people will have a fall because of decreased levels of activity, due to the pandemic.

Preventing the combination of disease and loss of fitness

The disease process can accelerate a person's rate of decline; for example, a heart attack will kill some heart muscle cells. For too many people, however, there is a greater acceleration of the rate of decline because they, and the people who care for them, assume that if you have a long-term health problem you should rest and do less. The good news is that even after the onset of disease, such as heart failure, the Fitness Gap can be closed by the 'Walking Plus' Programme, through not only walking but also daily exercises to increase skill, strength, and suppleness (see Chapter 1). This means that instead of dropping below 'The Line', becoming dependent on other people, and needing social care, a person who increases their level of physical activity after a diagnosis can become more able than they were before the onset of the disease.

Ludwig Wittgenstein, a great walker and philosopher, said that it should be possible to express every idea as a picture. In Figure 4 we show the 'picture' of the benefits of walking after the onset of a serious disease, when it is still possible to close the Fitness Gap and keep you above what we call 'The Line'. The Line is the level of ability necessary for vital tasks, such as getting to the toilet in time.

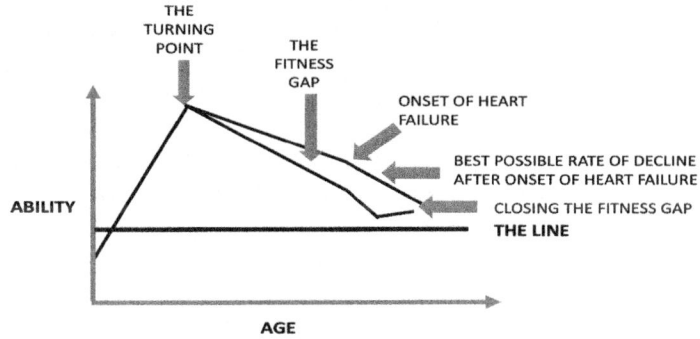

Figure 4: Closing The Fitness Gap after the onset of long-term conditions

How walking exerts its therapeutic effect

Walking sometimes affects the disease process directly, for example, by helping to reduce blood pressure in hypertension. But there are other beneficial effects of walking irrespective of a person's diagnosis:

- It reduces the levels of lipids and lipoproteins in the blood
- It reduces blood-sugar levels and, combined with dietary change, can cure Type 2 diabetes
- Many people who stop smoking find it easier to stay stopped if they also change their lifestyle. If, for example, the need for a cigarette is most strongly felt after a meal, why not walk 1,000 steps instead?
- It helps weight control and weight loss
- It reduces and prevents inflammation
- It increases mental wellbeing, particularly if joining a group, such as The Ramblers Wellbeing Walks

If you are worried about your condition, consult your doctor or nurse before increasing the amount you walk. The evidence is clear: if you have one or more long-term conditions, you have a greater need for walking briskly than people who do not have any. In addition, friends and family, or carers, who may feel happier pushing you in a wheelchair rather than lending you an arm and encouraging you to take extra steps, need a change of attitude. Some doctors are concerned about the risks of exercise. Although, when walking, there are a few risks that you need to minimise – cyclists on the pavement, for example (see Chapter 2) – the health risks from walking, including brisk walking, are greatly outweighed by the benefits. In 2021, in an important report from Sport England, the Royal College of General Practitioners, and the Medical Faculty of Sport and Exercise Medicine entitled *'Physical activity and health conditions; benefits outweigh risks'*, the emphasis throughout was that the benefits of physical activity outweigh risks.

Exercise will reduce the impact that disease has on your ability to look after yourself, which is why walking is now a type of therapy, promoted and prescribed by doctors, nurses, and the professionals who know most about disability – occupational therapists and physiotherapists (who can also advise on aids to help you with walking).

The benefits of exercise for the holistic care of all the major long-term conditions are now recognised and promoted by the charities representing people who have those conditions. The key facts about walking are presented in Chapter 9, which launches the 'BNWF' – the British National **Walking** Formulary – a new text to complement and supplement what every Doctor relies on – the BNF, the British National Formulary – listing the indications for, and dose of, every drug they can prescribe.

Remember you need to take action to increase all four aspects of fitness, strength, stamina, suppleness, and skill. Walking is very good for increasing stamina and strength of the leg muscles, so develop a daily programme of at least ten minutes to increase strength, skill, and suppleness.

We need a Walking Prescription linked to every prescription of a drug for a long-term condition.

CHAPTER 9

Walking prescriptions for common conditions

As well as concerns about the obesity epidemic, there is concern about the modern epidemics of cancer, Type 2 diabetes, dementia, and diseases of the heart and circulatory system. These epidemics have several causes, such as cigarette smoking and the modern diet. All these epidemics, however, result in part from physical inactivity. Type 2 diabetes, like obesity, can be regarded as a symptom of Walking Deficiency Syndrome, a condition not yet widely recognised by the medical profession.

Walking, often combined with other types of exercise, has been shown to be beneficial for all common long-term conditions. Some people with long-term health problems worry about taking more exercise, but none of the long-term health problems are exacerbated by walking.

The *British National Formulary*, or BNF, sometimes referred to as the Doctor's Bible, describes the correct drug formulation for all common conditions. As described in Chapter 8, it is now clear that walking is a therapy that also needs to be prescribed to help treat common long-term conditions, sometimes as well as, sometimes instead of, or before, drugs or psychological therapies are prescribed. The prescription of walking and other types of physical and social activities is known as 'social' prescribing or 'activity' prescribing. In this chapter, our focus is on prescribing walking using the BNWF, the British National **Walking** Formulary.

The origin of activity therapy

In 2016, the BBC made two TV programmes called *The Doctor Who Gave Up Drugs*, in which Dr Chris van Tulleken, now celebrated as the author of his book *Ultra-Processed People*, joined a general practice as a GP who was not able to prescribe drugs but could prescribe other treatments, usually involving other activities, but not drugs.

Some patients were resistant to this approach but other people were willing to stop taking prescribed drugs if they were to be supported in other activities, such as a walking group, an outdoor swimming club, or Kung Fu classes. Based on Dr van Tulleken's work, a new approach to medical practice, known as 'exercise therapy' or 'activity therapy', has evolved according to the following principles:

- Some people need only exercise therapy, not drug therapy
- Some people need exercise therapy before starting drug therapy, for example, a three-month training programme, with dietary change, before starting drug therapy for Type 2 diabetes
- All people with common long-term conditions who need drug therapy also need exercise therapy
- All people receiving psychological therapy should also be considered for walking therapy

Walking is the simplest type of activity therapy to prescribe or take.

Digital support for activity prescribing

The digital revolution in healthcare offers many opportunities for informing, enabling, and supporting people in taking more exercise and walking more.

Digital technology called W:ISH has been developed and approved to link data about a person's diagnosis, treatments, and postcode in their GP Record to local and online opportunities for becoming more active to the nearest Ramblers Wellbeing Walk for example, or to a gym where there is a programme for people with Type 2 diabetes. It will do this automatically, relying on the GP just to encourage the patient to become more active. The W:ISH system, however, will generate these activity prescriptions even if the GP forgets to do so, or is unaware of local opportunities.

Walking therapy for people with COPD (chronic obstructive pulmonary disease) and asthma

Breathlessness, or shortness of breath (dyspnoea), is a key symptom of the lung diseases COPD and asthma. The evidence shows that people with COPD or asthma need to focus on becoming fitter rather than avoiding getting breathless.

'Physical activity improves cardio-respiratory health. Furthermore, in COPD, exercise training reduces dyspnoea symptoms and increases ability for exertion.'

Exercise – the Miracle Cure.
Academy of Medical Royal Colleges, 2015

Brisk walking decreases breathlessness by helping the muscles become better at using oxygen in the bloodstream.

The charity *Asthma + Lung UK* has a major programme called Stay Active, Stay Well. Here, extracted and condensed, are some of the excellent tips and support the charity offers about keeping active with a lung condition, together with an outline of the range of activities suitable for someone with a lung condition.

'It's normal to get out of breath when you exercise. If you avoid activity that makes you get out of breath, this will make your breathlessness worse. Your muscles will get weaker and need more oxygen to work.

As your muscles recover after exercise, they adapt to use oxygen more efficiently. So, with regular exercise, you'll need to breathe less to do the same activity.

Over time, doing physical activity that makes you a little bit out of breath will help you feel less out of breath doing everyday activities. Physical activity includes walking, gardening and doing housework, as well as activities like swimming, playing sport and going to a gym.'

For people who have asthma, Asthma + Lung UK state that there are no bad activities, recommending:

- A daily walk
- Playing more vigorously with one's children and/or grandchildren
- Gardening
- Sitting down a little less each day

People with asthma who are in contact with Asthma + Lung UK

charity have provided feedback on how much they enjoy walking, especially with a walking group, because of the other benefits such as being outside in a green environment, and meeting people. They can also enjoy activities such as netball, or chair yoga, which are great for building confidence. There are a range of modified sports available, and you can search for inclusive sports groups in your local area.

It is important to bear in mind, however, that although brisk walking is a vital therapy for people with lung and breathing problems, if there is a Met Office warning of high levels of pollution, caution is necessary.

Walking therapy for people with heart disease

Angina is chest pain due to insufficient oxygen reaching the muscles of the heart. Some people develop angina and are diagnosed with heart disease when consulting their doctor about chest pain that typically occurs when exercising, but stops when at rest. It is a symptom of heart disease, but heart disease can come out of the blue, and the first sign that many people have is a heart attack. If you have angina, consult your doctor before increasing any type of activity.

There are now many effective treatments for angina and heart disease, but increasing activity is of great importance.

> *'All studies show clear improvements in cardio-vascular health with moderate exercise. There are similar beneficial effects for sufferers of angina. Overall, exercise reduces cardiac mortality by 31%.'*
>
> *Exercise – the Miracle Cure.*
> Academy of Medical Royal Colleges, 2015

The *British Heart Foundation*, the UK's leading heart disease charity, is committed to the promotion of exercise, including walking, and their website is full of information about the benefits of walking for people with heart disease. Among other high-value resources, the website provides:

- Top tips for summer walking

- Free walking apps
- Find a walking group

Hospital cardiology departments have also played a leading role in promoting the benefits of exercise for people with heart disease. It is now standard practice for a person who has had a heart attack, or who has had angioplasty and a stent inserted, to be referred to an exercise programme, including treadmill walking, to help them re-establish confidence and develop an exercise routine for their long-term health.

For people with heart failure, walking is an effective therapy because it helps to 'train' the muscles to extract more oxygen from the blood as it passes through them, independent of any weight loss that may occur.

Walking therapy for people with high blood pressure

People with high blood pressure (hypertension) are in greater need of walking therapy than people whose blood pressure is not high, as outlined in the Academy of Medical Royal Colleges report:

> *'Hypertension is responsible for 50% of strokes and 50% of ischaemic heart disease. Most people with hypertension are on long-term medication. Randomised controlled trials show a clear lowering of blood pressure with aerobic training. The scale of the reduction has been quantified: 31% of patients on average experience a drop of at least 10 mmHg with regular physical activity.'*

Exercise – the Miracle Cure.
Academy of Medical Royal Colleges, 2015

Walking reduces blood pressure not only directly, but also indirectly by helping to reduce a person's body weight. Obesity is a major cause of high blood pressure which, in turn, is a major cause of heart disease, stroke, and dementia.

Walking therapy for people with Type 1 diabetes

If you have diabetes, you have too much glucose in your blood. Glucose is a sugar that the body converts into energy, but if your sugar levels are too high, serious complications occur. There are two types of diabetes – Type 1 and Type 2.

Type 1 diabetes usually starts in adolescence, the cause of which is unknown. The body stops producing insulin, which is the hormone that controls blood-sugar levels. Unfortunately, the loss of insulin production cannot be reversed, so for the rest of their lives people who have Type 1 diabetes need to test and control their blood sugar several times a day by injecting insulin, or wearing an insulin pump.

For people with Type 1 diabetes, keeping fit and taking exercise, such as regular brisk walking, is vital because it reduces the amount of insulin the body requires and therefore the amount of insulin that needs to be injected. The Juvenile Diabetes Research Foundation UK (BreakthroughT1D) for young people with Type 1 diabetes, however, recognises that young people may need an activity more glamorous, vigorous, and anger-releasing than brisk walking, such as kickboxing or karate. Although walking briskly is a medium-intensity activity, young people with Type 1 diabetes also need to learn how to cope with the demands of the type of high-intensity activity that they will meet throughout the course of their lives, such as when dancing for an hour or doing high-intensity interval training (HIIT).

Walking therapy for people with Type 2 diabetes

In the UK, the number of people being diagnosed with Type 2 diabetes is rising dramatically. The condition starts gradually, and most commonly appears in people over 40 years of age. In Type 2 diabetes, the body often still produces insulin, but not in sufficient amounts to regulate blood-sugar levels, and so medication is usually prescribed. In some cases, insulin by injection also becomes necessary.

On its website, Diabetes UK highlights the fact that:

> *'Lots of people with Type 2 diabetes don't take any medication, and they instead treat their diabetes by eating well and moving more. Our latest research has even shown that weight loss can put Type 2 diabetes into remission.'*

Brisk walking will also reduce the risk of the complications of diabetes, such as heart disease or kidney failure, by lowering blood pressure and reducing cholesterol levels in the blood.

The Diabetes UK website lists the benefits of walking (see Box 10).

Box 10: The benefits of walking

- You can walk anywhere, any time, and it's free
- Walking briskly can help you build stamina, burn excess calories, and make your heart healthier
- It can help the body to use insulin more effectively
- It is easy on your joints
- It can benefit your mind by helping to reduce stress levels and symptoms of depression and anxiety

---

Walking should be prescribed as a therapy for everyone with Type 2 diabetes. Indeed, it should not only be prescribed but enabled, facilitated, and supported, for example by ensuring that everyone with Type 2 diabetes receives good-quality foot care known as podiatry. Podiatry is crucial for people with Type 2 diabetes, not only because of the importance of having healthy feet for walking well, but also to reduce the risk of the complications of Type 2, such as peripheral arteriopathy, which is damage to the blood vessels, and peripheral neuropathy, which is damage to the nerves, of the feet.

Walking therapy for people with arthritis

Versus Arthritis (www.versusarthritis.org) is a leading charity for people with arthritis. Although the organisation campaigns for better clinical care and for more resources for research, Versus Arthritis is also one of the organisations promoting walking as a therapy. One of the resources on its website, 'Top Tips for Walking with Arthritis', states that:

> *'Walking is recommended for people with arthritis as it is low impact, helps to keep the joints flexible, helps bone health, and reduces the risk of osteoporosis. If you do experience pain or you are very stiff afterwards, try doing a bit less, factor in more rest, and check in with your GP if you need to.'*

Versus Arthritis also provides guidance on how people with arthritis can start to increase the amount they walk over time (see Box 11).

Box 11: Versus Arthritis – Top Tips for Walking with Arthritis

Aim to start slowly with a manageable walk each day, thinking about what works with your daily routine. For example, moving around the house, walking the kids to school or arranging to walk with a friend.

1. Once you've got used to walking more regularly, you can choose to gradually lengthen your walks, or maybe you could walk a few more days each week.
2. Think about timing. Is first thing in the morning the best time for you or do you prefer a lunchtime walk?
3. Make your routes interesting and try urban and green space options depending on what's most accessible where you are.
4. Using crutches, walking poles or a stick can help with pain, balance and your posture.
5. You could try Nordic walking, it's very good exercise for the joints and by using poles you have extra support.
6. Alternatively, why not join a walking group? There's a range of organisations across the UK offering accessible walking sessions.
7. By adding a few stretching and strengthening exercises to your routine, this can help ease stiffness and strengthen your leg, back and core muscles. This is beneficial for everyday living, improving balance and walking.

Of the tips in Box 11, numbers 5 and 6 are specific for people with arthritis, whereas some of the other tips could apply to people who have other long-term conditions as well as to those with arthritis, such as tips 1-4 and 7.

Versus Arthritis also provides guidance on exercise for healthy joints.

Walking therapy for people with intermittent claudication

Intermittent claudication is muscle pain in the lower limbs, which occurs when people are active and stops when they are at rest. It is a symptom of peripheral arterial disease – the name given to the effects of the general condition called atherosclerosis, which affects the body's arteries, including those to the brain, heart, and lower limbs. In the lower limbs, atherosclerosis leads to a narrowing of the arteries and thereby a lack or insufficiency of oxygen-rich blood to the leg muscles which causes pain.

Brisk walking as therapy can increase the distance that people with intermittent claudication are able to walk before they need to stop due to pain, which is usually in the calf muscles.

> *'Exercise leads to a moderate improvement in peripheral vascular disease. Improvements are seen in both pain-free walking time, and distance, in several studies.'*
>
> *Exercise – the Miracle Cure.*
> Academy of Medical Royal Colleges, 2015

Walking as therapy for people with intermittent claudication increases the effectiveness of the muscles at extracting oxygen from the blood that flows through them, but walking does not help to open the narrowed blood vessels.

Walking therapy for people with osteoporosis

Osteoporosis is the thinning of bones, which makes them weaker and more fragile. This condition develops gradually, and often not diagnosed until someone has a fall that causes a bone to break, usually in the hip, wrist, or spine.

Osteoporosis can be delayed by walking, especially brisk walking, even in people with diseases that increase the rate of bone loss. In the *Physical Activity Guidelines* by the four Chief Medical Officers, to keep bones strong, people are encouraged not only to walk but to walk carrying heavy shopping. When bones are made to bear a load, it prevents bone thinning and helps to increase bone density.

The use of weights or kettlebells is also effective, and there is a good case for recommending weight training for all women. If you intend to start weight training, we recommend 1-2 sessions with a personal trainer or 1-2 classes at a fitness centre/gym to ensure you develop a good technique.

Walking, however, is crucial because the pressure it puts on the bones stimulates the strengthening of the bone tissue. The greater the amount of load-bearing work the bones have to do, the stronger they become.

Walking therapy for people with neurological disease – stroke, multiple sclerosis, and Parkinson's disease

A stroke is a life-threatening condition that occurs when the blood supply to part of the brain is cut off, which can lead to brain injury, disability, and death.

Walking reduces the risk of a stroke because it reduces blood pressure and the risk of atherosclerosis, the deposition of fatty material on the inner walls of the arteries ('furring').

The effects of a stroke may be minor in some people, and not last long, but for others the effects can be long-term and serious. Recovery of the ability to walk is a very high priority for stroke survivors, and the Stroke Association has a section on its website dedicated to 'Getting moving after a stroke', a 9-point list of suggestions. 'Moving More Every Day' is Point 3, which emphasises:

'You don't have to carry on for a long time. A ten-minute burst of activity several times a day can have the same benefit as a longer session.'

The Stroke Association provides several practical suggestions to encourage stroke survivors to move more (see Box 12).

> **Box 12: Moving more every day**
>
> - Try timing yourself doing the vacuuming, and try to beat your time another day. Put some music on while you're dusting to get you moving around the room.
> - Gardening tasks like weeding, digging and planting can build strength, and improve skills using hands and fingers.
> - If you can walk outdoors, it's a great way to get moving. You can build up the distance at your own pace and it's something you can do with a friend. You can add walking into your day by getting off the bus early, or walking to the shops instead of driving.
> - Climbing up stairs is a great way to get your heart working, as well as strengthening muscles. When you are out, try taking the stairs instead of a lift. Or try going up and down stairs in your home.

Multiple sclerosis (MS) is a lifelong condition affecting the brain and spinal cord. People with MS can have a range of symptoms, including problems with movement, sensation, or balance. A major focus is on retaining the skill of walking, both by prescribing the new disease-modifying drugs and by encouraging people to walk. Specific training programmes, designed to help people with MS overcome the particular and various obstacles experienced with this disease, are also important. The Multiple Sclerosis Society gives good advice on a range of activities people can do for themselves, including walking, highlighting how outdoor walking can improve balance. The Society recommends:

> *'If you're experiencing issues such as low mood, anxiety or depression, exercise may help you. Regular aerobic exercise has been shown to help relieve mild to moderate depression'.*

Parkinson's disease is a progressive condition in which parts of the brain become damaged. The main symptoms are shaking that the person is unable to control, slowness, and stiff or inflexible muscles. This combination of symptoms means that people with Parkinson's disease have problems with walking, particularly when they 'freeze' and are unable to take the next step.

Parkinson's UK, the leading charity for people with the disease, recommends walking as part of managing the symptoms, and specifically recommend a 'fast-paced 20-minute walk', particularly for people with progressing symptoms. Nordic walking is also featured as a suitable physical activity for people with Parkinson's disease. Walking, however, can present different challenges for different people with Parkinson's disease. For some, stiffness is the problem, but for others co-ordination may be difficult. The Parkinson's UK website has much useful information on how to tackle these challenges.

Sometimes a different approach is needed, and the benefits of dancing for people with Parkinson's disease are now well established. Indeed, dancing is a wonderful therapy for all long-term conditions, and walking plus dancing is a great combination for improved health and wellbeing.

Apart from these three common conditions, there are many other neurological conditions for which it is also important to help people regain, retain, and improve their ability to walk and thereby maintain social contact.

Walking therapy for people with cancer

Cancer is a condition where the body's cells divide and grow uncontrollably, causing a tumour to develop. The cells of some cancers can spread to other tissues in the body. Owing to advances in treatment – surgery, radiotherapy, and chemotherapy – and the possibility of cure for some cancers, cancer for many people is now considered to be a long-term condition.

Exercise should be prescribed for most people with cancer, and walking therapy can help as part of a programme of exercise. The charity Macmillan Cancer Support emphasises the importance of physical activity before, during, and after treatment for cancer. After treatment, Macmillan Cancer Support acknowledges the concerns people may have, but gives the following reassurance:

- *'You might be nervous about starting a physical activity plan, especially if you were not very active before your cancer treatment.*
- *You may worry that you are too tired or that you might*

injure yourself. But research shows that even a little activity is better than no activity at all. As you start to feel more confident, you can slowly build up the amount of physical activity you do.'

In addition, Macmillan Cancer Support emphasises that not only are there benefits from physical activity, but also most types of light physical activity, such as walking, are safe. It is noteworthy that someone had the vision and commitment to fund The Ramblers Association (as it was previously known) to launch the Walking For Health programme, after the Department of Health stopped funding Health Walks.

The Clinical Oncology Society of Australia has summarised the evidence-base on the benefits of exercise for people with cancer, before, during, and after treatment, in their 2018 position statement on exercise in cancer care:

'Clinical research has established exercise as a safe and effective intervention to counteract many of the adverse physical and psychological effects of cancer and its treatment. To date, the strongest evidence exists for improving physical function (including aerobic fitness, muscular strength and functional ability), attenuating cancer-related fatigue, alleviating psychological distress and improving quality of life across multiple general health and cancer-specific domains. Emerging evidence highlights that regular exercise before, during and/or following cancer treatment decreases the severity of other adverse side effects and is associated with reduced risk of developing new cancers and co-morbid conditions such as cardiovascular disease, diabetes and osteoporosis. Furthermore, epidemiological research suggests that being physically active provides a protective effect against cancer recurrence, cancer-specific mortality and all-cause mortality for some types of cancer (research has predominantly focused on breast, colorectal and prostate cancers).'

Exercise is also promoted by charities concerned with specific types of cancer. For instance, *Breast Cancer Now* has a web page titled 'Exercise during and after treatment'. Breast Cancer Now recommends shoulder and arm exercises to help regain the movement and function people had before surgery and/or radiotherapy, as well as other forms of exercise, as set out below.

Other exercise activities recommended for people undergoing various types of treatment for breast cancer

Type and phase of treatment for breast cancer	Other exercise activities apart from the shoulder and arm exercises after surgery, and/or radiotherapy
After surgery	• A short walk a few days after surgery; some people need longer to rest • Build physical activity levels up gradually
During and after chemotherapy	Gentle exercise such as walking
During and after radiotherapy	Gentle exercise that feels comfortable, such as walking, gentle stretching, Yoga, and Pilates
Taking hormone therapy	• Regular weight-bearing exercises • Regular pain relief and regular exercise, such as walking or swimming

Cancer care should include walking therapy as well as surgery, chemotherapy and radiotherapy.

Walking for people who are depressed and people who are anxious

Depression is a common mental health problem with people experiencing persistent sadness and a lack of interest in previously rewarding or enjoyable activities. Depression can disturb sleep and appetite; tiredness and poor concentration are common. The effects of depression can be long-term or recurrent, and affect people's ability to function and live a rewarding life. Depression can be prevented by physical activity. In the Academy of Medical Royal

Colleges 2015 report, *Exercise – the Miracle Cure*, it states that:

> *'There is a 20-33% lower risk of developing depression for adults participating in physical activity.'*

Physical activity can also be beneficial for people who have depression that requires some form of treatment. Although severe depression will need drug treatment, many people with depression and anxiety respond well to psychological therapies. A major NHS programme provides Independent Access to Psychological Therapies (IAPT) such as cognitive behavioural therapy (CBT) as an alternative to prescribing anti-depressants. There is increasing interest in complementing psychological therapies with prescribing physical activity.

Walking is one of the physical activities suggested by the charity *Rethink Mental Illness* that is considered to be beneficial for people's mental health and wellbeing through:

- the release of hormones called endorphins, which improve a person's mood
- increasing concentration
- improving sleep quality
- increasing confidence
- increasing motivation

Rethink Mental Illness is also delivering a Sport England-funded project called 'Rethink Activity' to help new and existing peer support groups introduce physical activity to their members to work towards being active for at least 30 minutes a week.

The benefits of walking in the countryside are also increasingly being recognised. The UK charity *Mind*, which is for anyone with a mental health problem, promotes the benefits of both formal and informal physical activity outdoors. On their 'Nature and Mental Health' web page, it states that:

> *'Spending time in green spaces, or bringing nature into your everyday life, can benefit both your mental and physical wellbeing, such as exercising outdoors.'*

The Mind website also has an informative section on Ecotherapy, defined as:

> '...a formal type of therapeutic treatment which involves doing outdoor activities in nature'

Research has shown that ecotherapy can help with mild to moderate depression. Ecotherapy can also be referred to as green exercise – exercising in green spaces, such as Ramblers Wellbeing Walks. A moving account of the benefits of walking, particularly walking in nature for people with depression, is given in the book by Isabel Hardman, entitled *The Natural Health Service.*

Walking therapy for people with severe mental health problems

Schizophrenia and bipolar disorder are often referred to as a severe mental illness. People with a severe mental illness have a significantly lower life expectancy than people who do not. There are many reasons for this, but one reason is the level of physical inactivity.

Most people with a severe mental illness like schizophrenia need drug treatment. But walking can play a part in their support, principally to help with managing weight gain, which is one of the common aspects of such conditions. Weight gain increases the risk of many other conditions that are more common in people with severe mental illness, as outlined in a 2018 report by Public Health England entitled *Severe mental illness and physical health inequalities.* People with these conditions have a higher prevalence of:

- Obesity
- Asthma
- Diabetes
- COPD
- Coronary heart disease
- Stroke
- Heart failure

Moreover, the report states that in England, people with severe mental illness:

- die on average 15-20 years earlier than the general population
- if under the age of 75 years, have a death rate 3.7 times higher than the death rate for the general population

Public Health England concluded that:

> *'SMI patients experience a higher prevalence of physical co-morbidities and multi-morbidities, and therefore there is a need for integrated and holistic care delivery which considers their mental and physical health needs.'*

The holistic care of people with severe mental illness should include interventions that encourage and enable physical activity. For people with severe mental illness who are living in a facility that lacks appropriate outdoor space, or who are not allowed outdoors for various reasons but whose needs are great, treadmills or exercise bikes with virtual reality, are stimulating and help to address levels of inactivity.

Walking for people affected by dementia

Dementia is a group of related symptoms associated with ongoing decline of brain functioning. There are many different types of dementia: Alzheimer's disease is one type, and together with vascular dementia, they comprise most of the cases.
Although in the past it was commonly thought the brain was an organ that did not change during adult life except to decline, research using remarkable new imaging equipment is changing our perceptions. In the Academy of Medical Royal Colleges report, *Exercise – the Miracle Cure*, it emphasises that:

> *'physical activity ... consistently reverses brain atrophy'.*

Therefore, walking can be beneficial for people affected by Alzheimer's disease or other forms of dementia. In the Alzheimer's Society leaflet 'Keeping active and involved', exercise is recommended for people's physical and emotional wellbeing, with walking suggested as a suitable physical activity as well as cycling, swimming, dancing, T'ai Chi, and Yoga.

If you care about, or for, a person with dementia, you could take them for a walk. There is a distinction to be drawn, however, between walking for exercise and 'walking about'. The website of the Alzheimer's Society explains this difference:

> *'Walking is not a problem in itself – it can help to relieve stress and boredom and is a good form of exercise. But as with all behaviour, if a person with dementia is walking about – and possibly leaving their home – it could be a sign that they have an unmet need. By understanding what they need and looking for solutions, you can help to improve their wellbeing.'*

The Alzheimer's Society is funding research into technological developments to address the common urge for people with dementia to walk about and possibly leave their home. There are also digital solutions, such as the MOTUS virtual reality system, which offers the opportunity for people with dementia to 'walk' in different and/or stimulating environments. For people with dementia who are not able to stand or walk, there is the option of making progress by sliding their feet back and forth on a plastic sensor while seated and receiving feedback on how far they have 'walked'.

Walking for people who want to increase their ability

We have emphasised that walking can prevent or reduce the loss of ability that affects people with long-term health problems. Many people have more than one problem, a condition sometimes called multimorbidity. People with more than one long-term problem who want to increase their ability can also benefit from walking more, although they may need help to do so.

There are many types of aid available. Physiotherapists and occupational therapists (OTs) are the key health service professionals when seeking advice about the most appropriate types of aid to suit people's needs. A walking stick reduces the risk of falling, but there is a range of walking aids that have wheels, and often a seat, which can help to transform a person's quality of life by increasing their mobility.

Social prescribing and the need for walking prescriptions

Although modern medical technology has had a considerable impact on population health through the diagnosis and treatment of acute and long-term conditions, it is not sufficient to improve people's health, wellbeing, and healthy life expectancy. According to The King's Fund website, social prescribing has been developed in recognition that:

> '... *people's health and wellbeing are determined mostly by a range of social, economic and environmental factors*'.

As such, social prescribing seeks to address people's needs in a holistic way. It also aims to support individuals to take greater control of their own health. Social prescribing can be used to support people:

- with one or more long-term conditions
- who need support with their mental health
- who are lonely or isolated
- who have complex social needs affecting their wellbeing

It is possible for social prescribing to be both personalised and localised because the GP record contains information, not only about an individual's age, diagnosis, and treatment, but also their postcode. The W:ISH system enables localisation, for instance, by introducing the person to a local Ramblers Wellbeing Walk, or to opportunities offered by local authorities, AgeUK, and the Active Partnerships of Sport England. The software also provides links to other digital opportunities, such as:

- the NHS Active 10 app, which measures brisk walking
- the relevant charity website
- EXi, an app for people with one or more long-term conditions, which analyses user health and fitness and prescribes a personalised physical activity programme.

Goldster, wellbeing service, provides a wide range of online classes and opportunities (www.goldster.co.uk).

This does not create extra work for the GP or practice nurse and because a reminder or nudge can be automatically linked to every repeat prescription and therefore create wonderful opportunities for pharmacies to sell trainers as well as perfumes.

Furthermore, people need to think not just about walking down a street or on a treadmill but about the many different types of walking that there are, which we summarise in Chapter 10 because you may want to try different types of walking.

CHAPTER 10

Try different types of walking

In this book so far, only one type of walking done at different speeds – regular and brisk – has been described, but there are many variants of walking you can try.

Talking walking

Intimacy is attractive. Sitting opposite someone over a coffee or a beer, face-to-face, eye-to-eye, may encourage the open exchange of information, but some people find it easier to talk and share confidences when eye contact is not possible, for example, when walking side-by-side.

> *'[Arthur Fletcher] caught [Emily Wharton] at last and forced her to come out with him into the grounds. He could tell his tale better, as he walked by her side, than sitting restlessly in a chair or moving awkwardly about the room on such an occasion, as he would be sure to do. Within four walls she could have some advantage over him. She could sit still and be dignified in her stillness. But in the open air, when they would both be on their legs, she might not be so powerful with him and he perhaps might be stronger with her.'*
>
> Anthony Trollope, The Prime Minister

Talking and walking is a nice thing to do, and different from the experience of sitting and talking. Why not try it? Next time someone drops in for a chat and coffee, suggest a walk as well.

Meeting walking

An increasing number of organisations are introducing walking meetings as well as standing meetings. Many people find it a more dynamic way to 'walk' through problems, find solutions, or coach peers, than sedentary, moribund, chair-based meetings.

In addition it is often good to do supervision walking, both the supervisor and the person being supervised may find difficult messages easier to transmit side by side rather than eye to eye.

Green walking

In 2007, the mental health charity 'Mind' published a fascinating report entitled *Ecotherapy: the Green Agenda for Mental Health*, in which the focus was the effect of green exercise on people with mental health problems. When a walk in a country park was compared with a walk in an indoor shopping centre, it was found that:

- 71% of participants reported decreased levels of depression after the green walk, whereas 22% felt their depression increased after walking through an indoor shopping centre, and only 45% experienced a decrease in depression
- 71% of participants said they felt less tense after the green walk, whereas 50% said their feelings of tension had increased after the shopping centre walk
- 90% of participants had increased self-esteem after the green walk, whereas 44% said their self-esteem decreased after window shopping in the shopping centre

In addition, from a survey of GPs working across England and Wales, 'Mind' found that over half agreed that ecotherapy is a valid and suitable treatment for anxiety (52%) and depression (51%).

The Centre for Sustainable Healthcare in Oxford has developed a major Green Health programme for people with mental health problems, including those who are most severely affected.

If a green walk can take place on rough ground, the benefit is even greater, as Scott Grafton emphasises in his book *Physical Intelligence*:

> *'Intense physical experience, particularly in complex natural settings, places demands on the brain to learn and be proactive, even as it refines action to allow for best performance.'*

In Japan, ecotherapy is sometimes known as 'forest bathing' or Shinrin-Yoku, described in the book the *Art and Science of Forest Bathing* by Dr Qing Li. Although Shinrin-Yoku is prescribed in Japan, there are opportunities for anyone to take advantage of this form of ecotherapy because of the effort that has been made to keep even small areas of wild, green space in the Japanese urban environment, however busy.

Awe walking

On the Psychology Today website, awe walking is defined as:

> *'... a stroll, in which you intentionally shift your attention outward instead of inward. So, you're not thinking about the tight deadline, the unfinished project, the strain in your relationship with your spouse, or concerns about the coronavirus.'*

There are several benefits from walking in awe-inspiring environments. In a study of 60 older adults, published in 2020 in the journal *Emotion*, half the participants were assigned to a group that went on 'awe' walks, and half were assigned to a group that went on 'simple' walks. People in the 'awe group' reported increasing experience of awe on their walks as the study went on, with a growing sense of wonder and appreciation for the details of the world around them. They also had significant boosts of positive emotions such as compassion and gratitude. In contrast, people in the simple-walk group tended to be more inwardly focused.

Silly walking

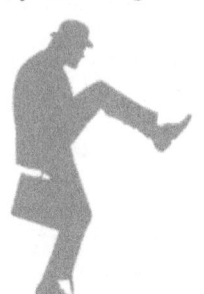

An article in the 2022 Christmas edition of the BMJ demonstrated the beneficial effects of walking like Mr Teabag (John Cleese) in the sketch in Monty Python's flying circus in the Ministry of Silly Walks. His style of walking is very inefficient, but can be classified as vigorous activity exercise!

Phoning walking

Phoning walking can assuage any feelings of guilt or pressure from a decision to walk for 30 minutes instead of taking a taxi or car to travel between meetings. If you are walking briskly, you may have to explain the reason for any heavy breathing to the person at the other end!

Reading walking

Reading while walking is not recommended when you are in a busy place like the High Street, or a beautiful place like the Cuillin Ridge! In quiet streets, it may pose less difficulties, although it is important to be aware of any uneven surfaces and other hazards on the pavement; for some people who have problems with walking, the average pavement now needs 100% concentration.

The combination of audio books, and other downloadable resources, and the smartphone, however, has the potential to transform walking from a physical exercise into a concert hall, a theatre, or book club. So, get walking, and listening!

Learning walking

In recent years, there has been an increasing emphasis on learning by listening, and as it is now possible to download podcasts and other educational resources onto smartphones, it is possible to listen and learn while walking. So get walking, listening, and learning!

Thinking walking

In a diatribe against walking, in 1918 Max Beerbohm reasoned:

> *'It rots the brain. Many a man has professed to me that his brain never works so well as when he is swinging along the high road, or over hill and dale. This boast is not confirmed by my memory of anybody who, on a Sunday morning, has forced me to partake of his adventure. Experience teaches me that whatever a fellow guest may have of power to instruct or to amuse when he is sitting in a chair, or standing on a hearth-rug, quickly leaves him when he takes one out for a walk.'*

This is only one opinion: the evidence from many sources is that walking aids thinking. The person who was arguably the best thinker of the 20th century, Ludwig Wittgenstein, moved from Cambridge to County Wicklow, partly because of the beauty of the countryside. His biographer, Ray Monk, writes that Wittgenstein took his notebooks with him on his walks in western Ireland and would often work outdoors. A neighbour reported that he once passed Wittgenstein sitting in a ditch, writing furiously, oblivious of anything going on around him. Other neighbours thought him mad and 'forbade him to walk on their land on the grounds that he would frighten the sheep' because he talked aloud to himself.

Immanuel Kant, philosopher and author of *The Critique of Pure Reason,* made walking around Königsberg his daily ritual. Kant was so regular in his time-keeping that the local Königsbergers could set their clocks by his peregrinations. Another philosopher who was even more reliant on walking was Friedrich Nietzsche, who loved walking in the Engadine in Switzerland, and wrote that he:

> *'Put no trust in any thought that is not born in the open, to the accompaniment of free bodily motion.'*

Sporty walking

Walking sports, such as Walking Football, Walking Tennis, and Walking Cricket, are increasing in popularity. It has been suggested that they could be called Renaissance sports because they offer rebirth to the sportsmen and women who thought their sporting days were over.

Mindful walking

Mindful walking combines movement and mindfulness, both of which are ways of reducing stress. The key is to empty your mind of worries about work or money and focus on your body and the environment. The 'Change to Chill' website provides six simple steps to help you practice mindful walking (see Box 13).

> **Box 13: Mindful walking**
>
> 1. Before beginning your walk, stand still for a few moments, focusing on your breathing. Take note of how your entire body is feeling
> 2. As you begin to walk, bring your full attention to the movements and sensations in your body
> 3. Notice the way you carry your body— the feelings in your feet, legs, arms, chest, and head
> 4. Once you have connected with the sensations in your body, begin to open your mind
> 5. If you find yourself distracted by other thoughts, simply return to the focus on the movements of your feet, your breath, or the sensations in your body
> 6. When you are done, notice how you feel.

'Slow Ways' walking

Slow Ways is a project to create a network of walking routes that connect Great Britain's towns, cities, and villages. Using existing footpaths, people will be able to use the Slow Ways routes to walk between neighbouring settlements or combine routes for long distance journeys.

Slow Ways walking encourages people to explore, find, and record walking routes between destinations:

- Have a look at their website which changes as people add more walks
- Put in your postcode and see what walks have been discovered and developed in your area; if there are no routes for the walk you want, the website tells you what you can do

Imaginary walking

Incarcerated in Spandau prison, Albert Speer had no pedometer, but he did have his shoe, with which he could measure both his stride and the circumference of the prison yard. Therefore, he was able to calculate how far he had crossed towards his notional destination –

Heidelberg, which was his birthplace, and 620 kilometres from Berlin – while circling the prison yard. It was, he wrote:

> *'....a training of the will, a battle against the endless boredom, but it is also the expression of the last remnants of my urge towards status and activity.'*

Albert Speer, quoted in Duncan Minshull,
While Wandering

Why not embark on an imaginary or remembered journey to give colour and romance to your daily walk to work? Try these examples:

- The West Highland Way from Milngavie (pronounced Milguy) to Fort William: 153 km
- Hadrian's Wall (Wallsend to Bowness on Solway): 135 km

Details of long walks can be found on The Ramblers website.

Virtual reality walking

The production of a virtual reality 'treadmill', by MotusVR Systems now offers people who are older, frail, and/or housebound the opportunity to walk safely along the West Highland Way or the Cornwall Coastal Path. With technology developed by MotusVR, the base is a solid platform that does not move, and there is a rail for the user to hold. A moving platform can unbalance even the most stable walker. Instead, the fixed platform detects the movement of a user's feet by means of special slippers, worn by the user, sliding forward and back.

Another MotusVR development is social virtual reality, where it is possible for several users – family, friends, or colleagues – to walk virtually in the same place, such as Paris or the Great Wall of China at the same time and to share the experience.

There is also a Motus Systems variant that allows a person who cannot walk, due to an inability to stand, to sit on a chair and slide their feet back and forth; the virtual reality recognises the distance they are covering and moves them forward, virtually. To their delight, people unable stand can progress a kilometre or two using this system.

Although the ideal is to encourage people to get out more, on days when it is not possible, virtual reality offers a stimulating alternative.

Race walking

> *'Race Walking is a progression of steps so taken that the walker makes contact with the ground, so that no visible (to the human eye) loss of contact occurs. The advancing leg shall be straightened (i.e. not bent at the knee) from the moment of first contact with the ground until the vertical upright position.'*
>
> Rule 230: Race Walking. International Association of Athletic Federations (IAAF)

Race walking is an Olympic sport, in which the judges watch for 'lifting' – whether the walker is not in constant contact with the ground – and knee bending, often a source of controversy. In making their decisions, judges must rely on 'the human eye' alone and, although competitors are barred by IAAF Rule 71 from wearing clothing that 'impedes the ability of the judge to observe the legs for straightness', judges' decisions are often contested. The movement in race walking looks unnatural, and the sport demands considerable commitment, not only because of the effort required but also because of the astonished or amused glances of onlookers when racing or when training on one's own!

Dog walking

In the Special Health Report 'Get Healthy, Get a Dog', Harvard Medical School recommends dog walking:

> *'If you're looking for a role model for a healthy lifestyle, look no further than your dog. Dogs naturally engage in healthy behaviors. They crave exercise and get excited by it. They sleep well and rest often. They love deeply and affectionately ... they subtly encourage us to want to live*

healthier — no nagging necessary... In one study comparing 536 dog owners with 380 non-owners, the dog owners were not only more likely to have healthier weights and to be more physically active, they were better from the point of view of blood pressure, high cholesterol, diabetes, and depression.'

Whether the person is walking the dog, or the dog is walking the person, the result is improved physical and mental health.

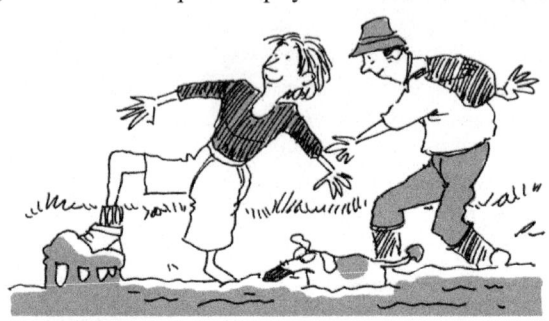

Wellbeing Walking

Finally, the Ramblers organise Wellbeing Walks. This is a vitally important service whereby trained volunteer leaders form groups for people who have lost confidence, to walk, can regain that confidence with great physical and mental benefits.

Purposeful walking

One of the features of Japanese life which makes it one of the populations in which people live longer better in good health is what they call Ikigai best translated as Purpose. Obviously walking to improve your health and increase the probability that you will live longer better is purposeful walking but even better is to have an altruistic purpose, one that will benefit others for example raising money for

- your local Wildlife Trust to improve the environment and save the planet
- the Royal Society for the Protection of Birds
- your local primary school's library

Walking briskly with purpose is even better than walking briskly so find a sponsor and raise money for other people.

CHAPTER 11

Generating political action for the walking revolution

This book has been written to help people walk more during their daily life.

Opportunities for a change in lifestyle, however, must not be left solely to the initiative of individuals. Social action can facilitate and motivate individuals, but social action requires political will. Politicians are becoming more aware of the growing problem posed by a culture of car dependency and the potential for promoting wellbeing through active travel. One of the unintentional benefits of the Covid pandemic, particularly during periods of lockdown, was an increased focus on walking and cycling as exercise.

Political action is necessary, not only to improve the facilities for individual walkers and local communities, but also to help the planet by reducing carbon emissions, especially through reducing car dependency and increasing active travel such as cycling and walking. But there is no point simply blaming people for having the wrong lifestyle. We have to recognise we are facing a new environmental challenge.

The new environmental challenge

In the 19th century, communicable disease epidemics were caused by the environment in which people lived, for instance, the spread of cholera through contaminated water. It was not possible for individuals to protect themselves. Instead, large-scale engineering schemes to provide clean water were needed, which in turn required a society wealthy enough to pay for such schemes, and equipped with the political capacity to make the change happen.

Epidemics of the 21st century, such as the obesity or Type 2 diabetes epidemic, are more complex. Their origins were initially identified as problems of lifestyle and personal choice, and the key intervention to tackle them was seen as giving information and educating people about healthier choices.

For some health problems, such as the effects of cigarette smoking – although the cause and effect are directly related and an individual may have some control over their behaviour – political action also has an important role in controlling the advertising of, or increasing taxation on, tobacco products. Other health problems, such as inactivity, are more complex and although they are often perceived as 'lifestyle' problems it is better to think of them as environmental problems. Although the evidence of harm is as equally strong as that on the harmful impacts of cigarette smoking, the change in behaviour required is influenced by many factors outside of an individual's control, such as:

- Urban planning that has encouraged 'urban sprawl'
- The development of out-of-town shopping and the closure of local shops
- Under-investment in public transport and investment in roads

All these factors result in increasing car ownership among people in more affluent areas.

In 2016, *The Lancet*, one of the most prestigious medical journals in the world, published a series of papers on urban design and health. The main conclusions were:

- *Land use and transport policies contribute to worldwide epidemics of infections and non-communicable disease through traffic exposure, noise, pollution, social isolation, low physical activity, and sedentary behaviours*
- *Policies need to ensure the provision of a safe walking and cycling infrastructure*

The aim is to increase the 'walkability' of the environment, but what is it that makes one environment more walkable than another? The presence of relatively large, safe, green spaces such as parks, is important, but research findings demonstrate that even small green spaces, such as 'parklets', encourage people to walk in their local environment.

In Scotland, the organisation that promotes walking, *Paths for All*, undertook a survey in 2019, which revealed that:

- While 41% of Scots agreed that pavements in their local area are in a good condition, almost as many (37%) disagreed.
- The majority of Scots (63%) had recently experienced problems that forced them to change their walking route or made them less likely to walk in the same place in future. The most common issues were cars parked on pavements, cyclists on pavements, and poor pavement maintenance.

In England, *Sustrans*, whose mission is to promote and facilitate cycling and walking, produced a report in 2021 on the changes people identified that would increase the 'liveability' of their environment. Of the people surveyed, 66% supported, while 12% opposed, the creation of more low traffic neighbourhoods. However, LTNs (Low Traffic Neighbourhoods) have become a political hot potato, more because of the restriction on driving than because of anything to do with walking.

In a major report by S. Claris and D. Scopelliti of the engineering company ARUP, entitled Cities Alive: Towards a Walking World, the benefits of walkability and the way to achieve them were described as follows

> *'We need to design physical activity back in to our everyday lives by incentivising and facilitating walking as a regular daily mode of transport. In addition to the host of health benefits, there are many economic benefits for developers, employers and retailers when it comes to walking. It is the lowest carbon, least polluting, cheapest and most reliable form of transport, and is also a great social leveller. Having people walking through urban spaces makes the spaces safer for others and, best of all, it makes people happy.'*

The 'social' engineering aim is to increase the 'walkability' of the environment, but what is it that makes one environment more walkable than another? In 2006, in an important article by Maria Creatore and colleagues on the 'Association of Neighborhood Walkability with Change in Overweight, Obesity, and Diabetes', published in The Journal of the American Medical Association, they defined criteria that could be used to assess the walkability of a neighbourhood (see Box 14).

> **Box 14: Criteria to assess the walkability of a neighbourhood**
>
> 1. Population density – number of people per square kilometre
> 2. Residential density – number of occupied residential dwellings per square kilometre
> 3. Number of walkable destinations – retail stores, schools, and services such as libraries, banks, and community centres within a 10-minute walk
> 4. Degree of street connectivity – number of intersections with at least three converging roads or pathways

There is, however, a fifth criterion that should be added to this list: the availability of good-quality green and blue space in the environment. The presence of relatively large, safe green spaces, such as parks, is important, but research findings demonstrate that even small green spaces, such as 'parklets', are important in encouraging people to walk in their local environment.

Mobilising political action

For the UK

In 2017, the UK Department for Transport published a 'Cycling and Walking Investment Strategy', in which the Government wants:

> *'to make cycling and walking the natural choice for shorter journeys and as part of a longer journey'*

The goals of this strategy are:

> *'By 2040 our ambition is to deliver:*
>
> *BETTER SAFETY*
>
> - *reduced community severance*
> - *streets where cyclists and walkers feel they belong and are safe*
> - *safer traffic speeds, with 20 mph limits where appropriate*

BETTER MOBILITY

- *urban areas that are considered as amongst the most walkable globally*
- *dense networks of routes around public transport hubs and town centres, with safe paths along busy roads*
- *better links to schools and workplaces*
- *technological innovations which promote walking and cycling*

BETTER STREETS

- *places designed for people, with walking and cycling put first*
- *a wider green network of walkways, cycleways and open spaces that let people actively incorporate nature into their daily lives'*

In January 2022, the Government announced the launch of Active Travel England (ATE), a new agency which builds on the Government's commitment to boost cycling and walking, and deliver a healthy, safe, and carbon-neutral transport system. Chris Boardman, the Olympic gold medal-winning cyclist, was appointed as the first Active Travel Commissioner for England to spearhead the establishment of the agency.

For London

It is possible to generate change at a local level much more quickly than it is at a national level. For example, the Mayor of London, together with Transport for London (TfL), is taking a 'Healthy Streets' approach to help Londoners use cars less, and walk, cycle, and use public transport more, using 10 Healthy Streets indicators (see Box 15).

> **Box 15: Transport for London's 'Healthy Streets' indicators**
>
> 1. Pedestrians from all walks of life
> 2. Easy to cross
> 3. Shade and shelter
> 4. Places to stop and rest
> 5. Not too noisy
> 6. People choose to walk, cycle, and use public transport
> 7. People feel safe
> 8. Things to see and do
> 9. People feel relaxed
> 10. Clean Air

Transport for London has acknowledged a responsibility towards increasing the number of people who walk in and around London. It has set up an excellent webpage on walking with a variety of resources such as:

- walking routes of less than 20 minutes in central London, and walking routes in the City of London
- family-friendly nature walks, and London nature trails
- maps of station-to-station walking steps and times in central London

For Manchester

In 2017, the Greater Manchester Combined Authority (www.greatermanchester-ca.gov.uk) launched a 'Greater Manchester Moving' (GM Moving) plan, renewed in the light of the impact of the Covid pandemic, aimed at making:

> *'Everyone in Greater Manchester more active, to secure the fastest and greatest improvement to the health, wealth and wellbeing of the 2.8 million people of Greater Manchester.'*

For your neighbourhood

Political change, however, needs to be driven by a range of inputs, including people like you, dear reader. Many more people who do not see themselves as lobbyists or pressure-group members could take action. Make an appointment to see your MP at their weekly surgery, even if your MP has never expressed an interest in walking or in how your city could be changed to encourage walking. If a sizeable number of MPs understood the need for change and said as much to the Ministers responsible, the impact would be considerable. If we want political action, it is up to us, the people who walk, to become political.

As long ago as 2012, the National Institute of Health and Care Excellence (NICE) issued strong, clear public health guidance with the title 'Physical Activity: walking and cycling'. The NHS and local authorities need to follow the guidance and take action, such as the examples below:

- Bus companies could show the distance between bus stops at every stop to encourage people to get off 2 stops early, and walk
- Every person with a long-term health problem needs a walking prescription together with, and sometimes instead of, a drug prescription, as well as advice on how to increase the amount they walk each day, including information about Wellbeing Walks
- Pavements need repair and improvement with benches at intervals to encourage urban walking
- There needs to be urban planting of, and caring for, trees to create mini forests and green paths

Walking can transform the health of individuals, communities, and populations. It can also contribute to reducing global climate change, but both require political commitment, support, and action. It is time for the Walking Revolution, and there are four Charities which are leading the revolution - the Ramblers, Sustrans, Living Streets and Parkrun.

The Ramblers

The Ramblers were formed in 1935, following three years in which there had been a growing resistance to the privatisation of the ancient Commons, some landowners blocking traditional Rights of Way. The need for an such an organisation continues but the Ramblers, and its Scottish equivalent Paths for All, do much more than this. The members of the Ramblers maintain and improve footpaths, repair stiles and gates and, most important of all, organise walks. These walks are enjoyed by many of the 100,000 Ramblers members, but of particular importance are the Wellbeing Walks. These help people recovering from illness to regain the ability and confidence to join Ramblers in all the walks that are available locally, and to build walking into their daily life.

Sustrans

The mission of Sustrans is to 'make it easier for everyone to walk and cycle'. To do this they have a wide range of activities designed to make cycling and walking not only easier and more enjoyable, but also safer. This includes measures to reduce traffic speed and volume, and better connection of people to green spaces and safe paths. They are influential with Local Authorities and persuade them to think of 'Transport' not simply as being about cars and buses but also about people and wellbeing. Sustrans has a very good grip of national transport policy issues and plays an important part in influencing policy to create walkable neighbourhoods for everyone, no matter what their level of ability.

Living Streets

The mission of Living Streets is to 'make streets better for walking' and they have number of workstreams to achieve this objective. They are working to make walking in towns easier, for example by improving pavements to reduce 'Slips, trips and falls', and reducing car parking on pavements. They encourage the authorities to put in more crossings for people on foot and to slow the traffic and they campaign to make walking safer by reducing both air pollution and the fear of crime. They promote the needs of people who rely on wheelchairs to get about and have a major focus on walking to school, and with many successes in getting the pupils excited and involved in campaigns to qualify for the WOW badge.

Parkrun

This has been a revolutionary movement in the last decade with weekly 5K runs in a local park, but it is very clear that you can walk as well as run and parkwalk now has a clear brand of its own. New digital technology will ensure that patients are informed about their nearest parkrun and parkwalk without the GP having to know or do anything other than give encouragement.

Take action to increase your wellbeing

The NHS remains vitally important for the diagnosis of disease and starting the right treatment. However, for disease prevention, adapting to long-term conditions, and feeling well, much more is needed. The World Health Organisation emphasises that health and wellbeing is much more than the absence of disease. Walking – particularly in a green environment – reduces the risk of disease, complements and supplements the benefits of high-tech medicine if disease has developed, and helps you feel and function better.

The last fifty years have seen our environment dominated by the car and we need a revolution to create or re-create an environment for walking well and safely. Working in a group for a good cause, such as the promotion of walking with these charities, is also good for your own wellbeing and will reduce the risk of dementia by strengthening your sense of purpose, or Ikigai, as the Japanese call it.

The time is right for the Walking Revolution, so let's get going!

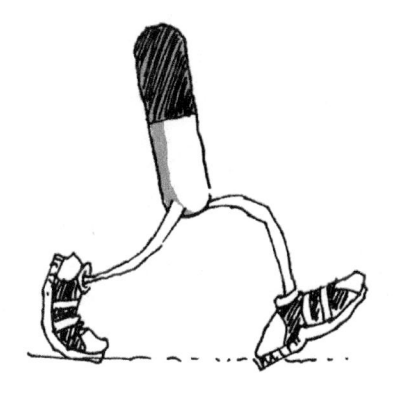

Websites of great organisations supporting walking

When you take a pill you can be sure that there is an industry behind it, not just a factory but research workers, regulators, pharmacies and many others, not to mention the doctor who prescribed the pill. It is the same with walking. There are many organisations which promote and facilitate walking and some of these are local branches of the national organisations listed below.

To start, just type into Google the name of your town or postcode along with the words 'health walks' and hit the button. Obviously the results vary from place to place but there are always health walks, with a leader, usually organised by

- Your local council
- The Ramblers
- The local 'branch' of Sport England, called an Active Partnership
- Local community centres and faith organisations
- The local Wildlife Trust

Active 10 is an app produced by the NHS to promote exercise. It measures how many minutes of your walking are brisk. We owe a lot to national charities which are committed to improving the environment and encouraging walking, and here are the key organisations.

Age UK organises walks for fundraising but it also promotes the benefits of walking for people who have already developed long-term health problems and has a very useful web page on walking tips and advice for older people. It also plays a leading part in promoting walking football, and more recently walking tennis.

Alzheimer's Society organise Memory Walks, not only for fund-raising but also because of the importance of walking and memories for people with dementia.

Asthma and Lung UK organises a number of different walking challenges such as a 10,000 steps challenge and a mountain trek challenge, not only for fundraising but to promote the benefits of walking.

Breast Cancer UK promotes walking as a factor which can reduce cancer risk.

Breast Cancer Now promotes a range of walks including Pink walks for fundraising, to promote health and reduce the risk of disease.

British Heart Foundation supports and promotes a wide range of different types of walking, not only to reduce the risk of heart disease but also to improve the function of the heart for people with heart disease, and their Heart Matters Walking is a major campaign.

Centre for Ageing Better not only runs a major campaign against ageism but also promotes Age Friendly Communities. As part of this has developed a method for doing Walk Audits to assess the walkability of a neighbourhood.

Centre for Sustainable Healthcare has a major green therapy programme including Green Walking for people recovering from mental health problems.

Country Walking is a very well produced monthly walking magazine, digital and paper, allowing you to experience many walks you will never be able to do. They also organise a great challenge you can join called Walk 1000 miles.

Diabetes UK organises many walks for fundraising, including KiltWalks in Scotland! It also emphasises the therapeutic benefits of walking for both Type 1 and Type 2 diabetes. They have succeeded in changing the culture of management of Type 2 diabetes so that walking is seen as an integral part of therapy.
Intelligent Health mobilises communities to take action to improve their health and wellbeing and one of their programmes is Beat the Streets, which incentivises people of all ages, particularly school children to walk more.

Living Streets does great work, particularly in cities, to increase walkability and is running a strong campaign against Pavement Parking.

Macmillan Cancer Support encourages a wide variety of different types of walks, including their Mighty Hikes and provides good advice on training for walking more. They also play a vitally important part in developing Wellbeing Walks because they sponsored the first three years of these walks, organised by the Ramblers, after the Department of Health stopped funding them.

MIND promotes walking for fundraising and emphasises the benefits of walking with nature.

Pacer is a very clever website allowing you to find easy walks near you. It also has a useful pedometer App.

Parkrun which is sponsored by Vitality is an organisation which not only stimulates hundreds of thousands of people to run or walk in a parkrun or parkwalk but also engages thousands of volunteers each week in organising the local walks.

Paths for all is the key organisation leading the development of active transport in Scotland, including Health Walks and promoting the benefits of walking for people with serious health problems like cancer and dementia.

Ramblings on BBC TV hosted by Clare Balding is helping people understand the emotional and existential importance of walking; it is the optimal wellbeing service, particularly walking in a green environment as Kathy Willis describes in her book *Good Nature*.

Rethink Mental Illness organises a wide range of walks, partly for fundraising but also for the benefit that walking brings for mental wellbeing as well as physical wellbeing, including for people who already have severe problems. For example, their Wild Ways for Wellbeing Walks emphasises the benefits of nature for people with mental health problems.

Royal Voluntary Service has a major Step Up campaign encouraging people to walk and run for their wellbeing, and to raise funds for local initiatives.

Slow Ways is developing a map of ways of walking from town to town and has produced a great *Sloways Pocket Atlas* showing 9,000 routes between towns and villages, all of which can be seen in more detail on their website.

Stroke Association promotes walking, not just for fundraising but for its benefits, particularly in reducing the risk of stroke as well as promoting walking and other types of exercise for people who have had a stroke.

Sustrans works tirelessly to influence transport policy in favour of walking and cycling.

The National Trust sees walking as a way of increasing wellbeing while enjoying the majesty of its properties and places.

The Parkinson's Society promotes walking especially for people with the condition because 'it has an impact both physically and mentally and can help manage Parkinson's symptoms.'

The Ramblers campaigns for walkers and organises a huge range of walks including Wellbeing Walks which are specifically designed for people with health problems and are a very important activity therapy service. Paths for All is the equivalent organisation in Scotland promoting Walking for Health, and organising Health Walks. Ramblers members receive their excellent magazine called *Walk*.

The Richmond Group co-ordinates the work of charities focused on specific health problems, and the work being done on walking by these charities is of great importance in the development of walking therapy.

The Wildlife Trust promotes walking emphasising the benefits of green walking and its book *Wildlife Walks* highlights 475 wonderful walks.

Versus Arthritis has developed walking groups for people with arthritis and plays a major role in promoting walking as a therapy, including research programmes such as Walk with Ease.

To access these resources please visit our website where we provide links to all the organisations websites.

www.drgrayswalkingcure.net/resources

Printed in Dunstable, United Kingdom